Meal Prep for Weight Loss

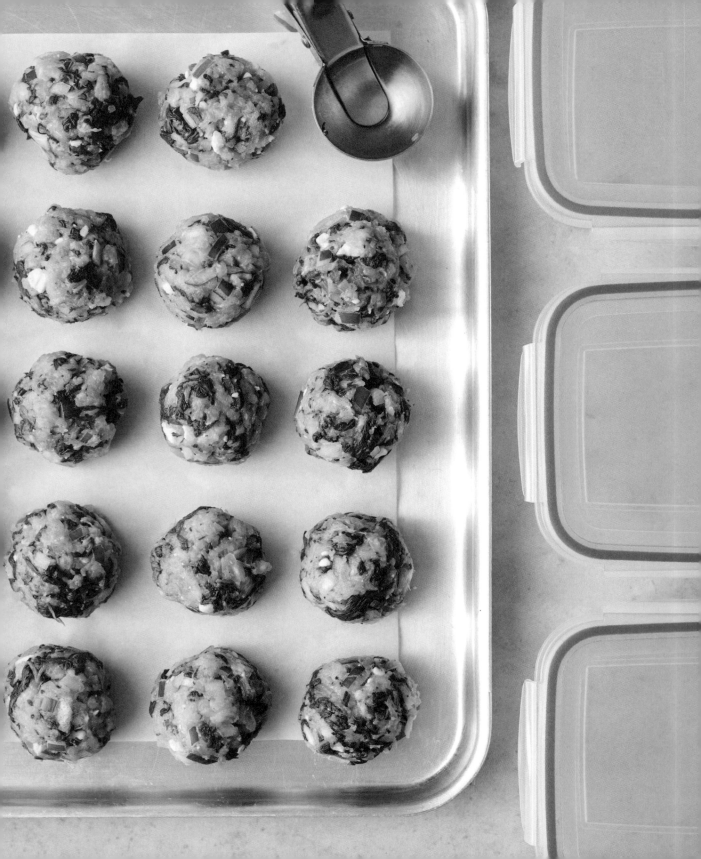

MEAL PREP
for weight loss

WEEKLY PLANS AND RECIPES TO LOSE WEIGHT THE HEALTHY WAY

Kelli Shallal, MPH, RD, CPT

Photography by Darren Muir

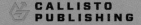

CALLISTO PUBLISHING

Published by Callisto Publishing LLC C/O Sourcebooks LLC
P.O. Box 4410, Naperville, Illinois 60567-4410
(630) 961-3900
callistopublishing.com

Printed and bound in China.
1010 24

*In memory of my grandparents,
Betty and Kenneth Hobby, for teaching
me that everything is possible, especially
the impossible.*

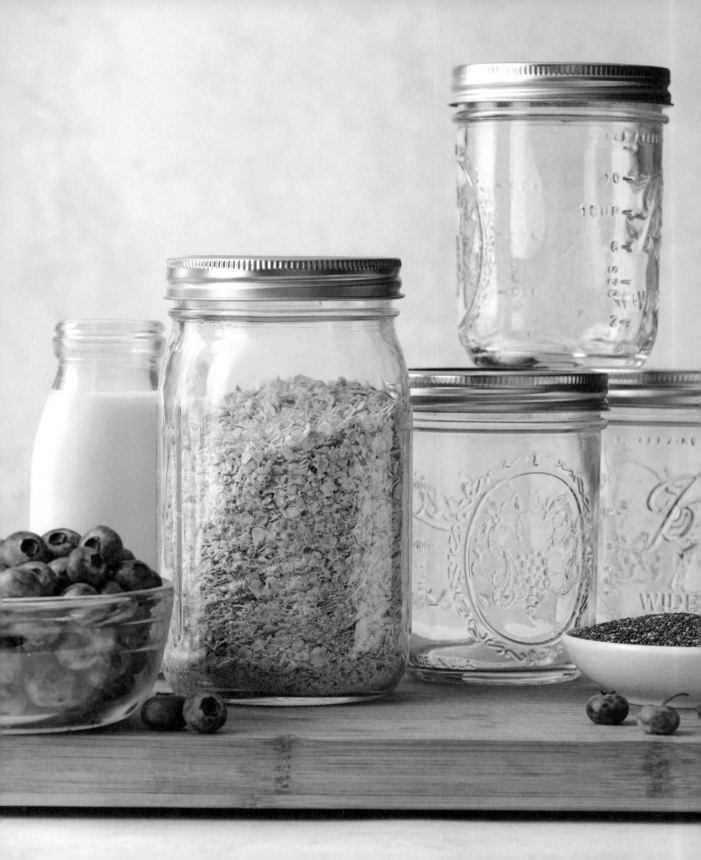

Contents

Introduction viii

PART ONE: MEAL PREPPING FOR WEIGHT LOSS

CHAPTER ONE **How to Lose Weight** 3

CHAPTER TWO **How to Meal Prep for Weight Loss** 13

PART TWO: WEIGHT LOSS MEAL PREP PLANS WITH RECIPES

CHAPTER THREE **Basic Three-Recipe Meal Preps** 29

CHAPTER FOUR **Batch-Friendly Four-Recipe Meal Preps** 45

CHAPTER FIVE **Flavor Variety Five-Recipe Meal Preps** 63

CHAPTER SIX **Superefficient Six-Recipe Meal Preps** 87

PART THREE: BATCH-FRIENDLY RECIPES

CHAPTER SEVEN **Healthy Carb Recipes** 113

CHAPTER EIGHT **Delicious and Healthy Veggies** 129

CHAPTER NINE **Satisfying Proteins** 143

CHAPTER TEN **Snacks** 157

The Dirty Dozen™ and the Clean Fifteen™ 169

Measurement Conversions 170

Index 171

Introduction

As a registered dietitian and personal trainer, I've always appreciated meal prepping as a strategy for maintaining good health. It wasn't until I became a new mom, however, that I truly fell in love with meal prep. Before the birth of my son, I prepared 25 healthy freezer meals that truly saved us during the early days having a newborn. When those meals ran out, I quickly realized that if I didn't prep full meals, I would subsist on whatever was closest and immediately available.

When my son grew older, I went back to work and things never slowed down. Instead, they only got busier as he became more active. Meal prep was the only way I was able to lose the 40 pounds I put on during pregnancy. (I know, I know. I'm a dietitian—didn't I know better? Well, dietitians aren't immune from weight gain and the only thing that made my nearly 30 weeks of nausea subside was bread and cheese.)

If you're reading this book, like many of my clients, you've probably tried to lose weight many times. The average American starts a new diet six times a year. The diet industry is a multi-billion-dollar industry for a reason. It preys on your deepest hopes and fears. It wants you to believe that quick and fast weight loss is the best way to get results. The truth is, sustainable weight loss is slow and steady. It requires significant lifestyle changes, as well as learning how to cook nutritionally balanced meals. There are no quick fixes in this book but, using meal prep, I will teach you the skills and nutrition knowledge to be able to lose weight sustainably and keep it off successfully.

This book includes a range of weekly meal prep plans, from basic three-recipe meal prep plans to superefficient six-recipe meal prep plans. Each meal prep plan provides everything you need to execute an effective meal plan for healthy weight loss. Recipes are both healthy and tasty, and the majority are in line with the Mediterranean or DASH diet guidelines. Meal prep plans include shopping lists as well as step-by-step cooking lists. Portioning, storing, and reheating instructions are included as well. You'll have everything you need to make losing weight easier and hassle free. So, let's get started!

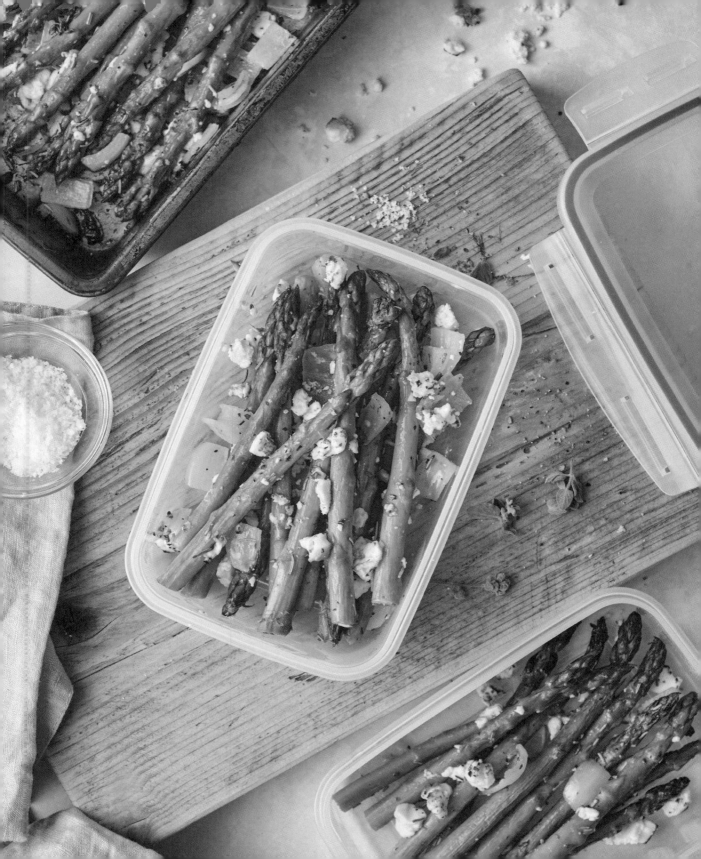

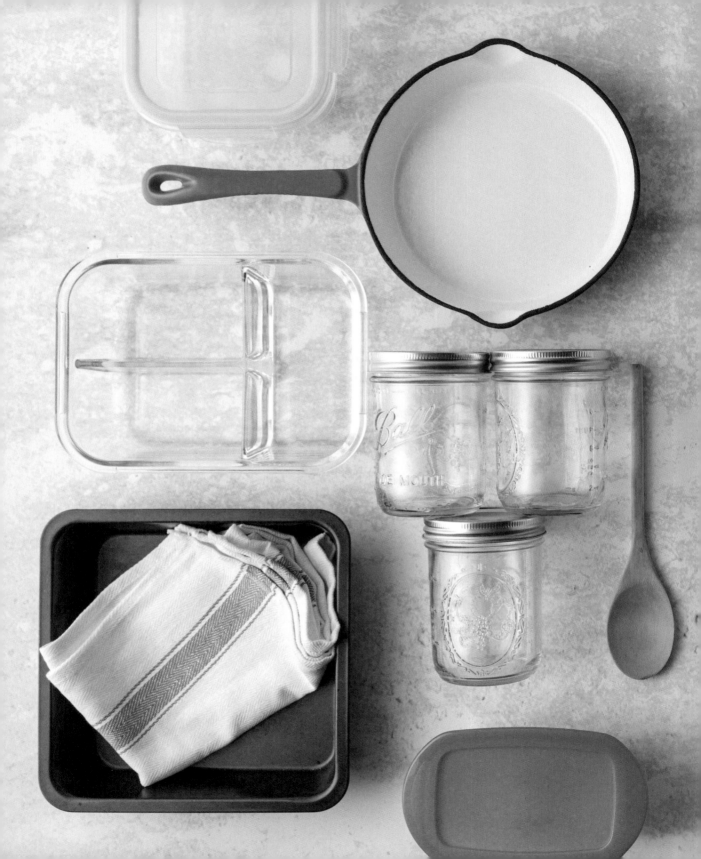

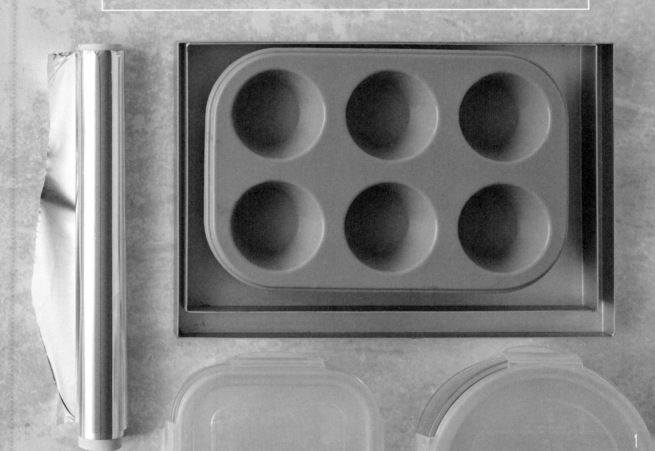

PART ONE

MEAL PREPPING
for Weight Loss

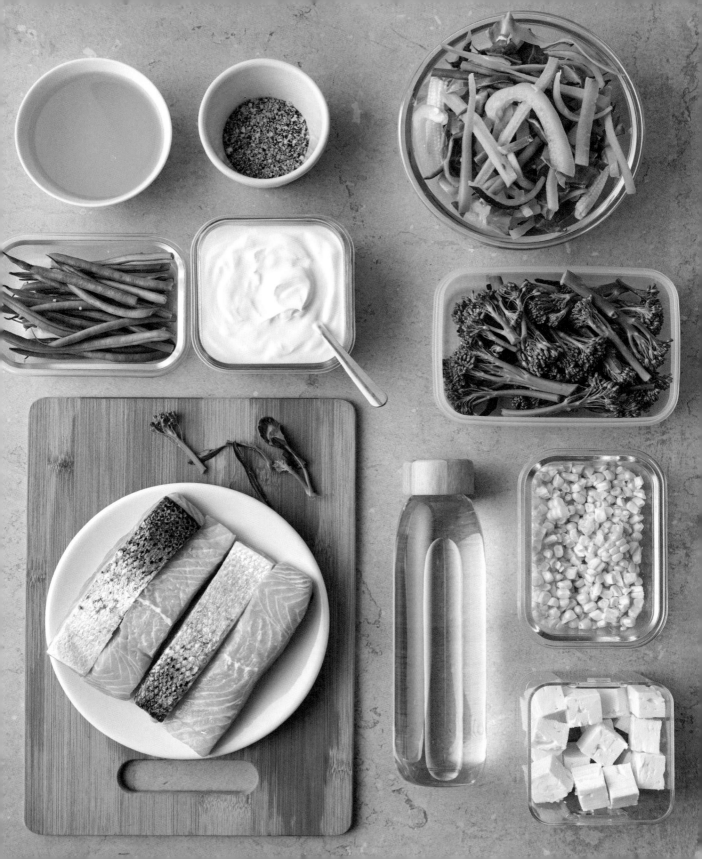

CHAPTER ONE

How to Lose Weight

This chapter reviews some basic concepts necessary for losing weight successfully through meal prep. It also details the nutritional foundation used to set up the meal plans and recipes. The goal is to equip you for long-term success when you are no longer relying on the provided plans and meal prepping your own meals.

A Healthy Approach to Weight Loss

For most people, the healthiest approach to weight loss starts with a major shift in their mind-set and lifestyle. I recommend eliminating the word "diet" from your vocabulary and never using it again. Instead, focus on creating a healthy lifestyle that allows some flexibility for special occasions.

Once you've set your mind to improving your health, you're ready to take action. The approach I lay out in this book is intended to help you create a healthy lifestyle that facilitates weight loss. If you can eat healthy 80 percent of the time, you will still be able to lose weight and enjoy treats the other 20 percent of the time. Meal prepping is a powerful tool to help you reach that 80 percent because it creates consistency in your eating behavior. This consistency leads to long-term lifestyle change instead of a (temporary) quick fix.

A REVIEW OF THE BASICS

In this book we will use the "plate method," the method I teach all of my nutrition clients. It does not require you to count calories, weigh your food, or agonize about anything. Instead, the plate method empowers you with the basics of healthy eating and a strategy to build a meal that will promote weight loss and weight maintenance.

The plate method consists of balancing the amount of protein, fat, carbohydrates, and fiber in every meal to promote a steady energy level and fat loss. Every time you put together a meal, it should follow these general guidelines:

- Fill half your plate with veggies.

- Fill the other half of your plate with a combination of healthy fats, lean proteins, and high-quality carbohydrates.

Portion specifics are provided later but, for now, keep this general setup in mind as your ticket to weight loss.

If you choose to count calories or macros (grams of fat, carbs, and protein), you'll learn how to calculate and customize them to your needs on page 9. Before we get into the nitty-gritty, though, there are a few important factors—such as calories, activity levels, and genetics—we need to discuss first.

CALORIES IN, ENERGY OUT

You are probably familiar with the concept that you need to burn more calories than you take in to lose weight. You may have heard the phrase "eat less and move more." However, I find that most of my clients don't eat enough—at least not enough of the right foods. Most people don't need to eat less but, rather, they need to change what they eat. You can eat far more protein and produce for far fewer calories and be much fuller than if you ate the same number of calories in fat and processed foods.

The mistake that the majority of dieters make is that they create too big of a deficit in calories too fast. When a huge calorie deficit is created to achieve weight loss for a sustained period, the body enters starvation mode and works to conserve every calorie consumed by lowering its resting metabolic rate.

A resting metabolic rate, or RMR, is the number of calories used in functions such as pumping the heart and breathing, tasks that keep you alive even if you were lying in bed all day. Think of your RMR like a thermostat. You can turn it up or down depending on several factors. Eating under your baseline needs will lower it, so you need to eat at or above this number to keep it from lowering itself. Have you ever wondered why many people who lose weight gain it back? It's because they eat under their RMR requirements, which lowers their metabolic rate.

For example, let's say someone has an RMR of 1,500, and goes on a long-term 1,200-calorie diet. Because they're not meeting the body's baseline caloric needs to cover basic bodily functions, the body thinks it is starving, and lowers its RMR to 1,200. After they have lost the desired weight and go back to regular eating, this dieter needs to eat 300 fewer calories just to maintain the weight. This isn't a lot in a day but, over the course of a week or a month, it becomes significant and leads to weight gain rather than maintenance.

If you make sure you always eat above your resting metabolic rate and aim for slow weight loss (between ½ pound and 2 pounds per week), you will not fall victim to a lowered metabolic rate. With that said, to lose weight and keep it off, you should be calorie conscious but not take it to the extreme. You can, however, safely increase your rate of weight loss by adding more exercise to create a more significant calorie deficit between your total daily expenditure and your resting metabolic rate needs.

SEDENTARY VERSUS ACTIVE LIFESTYLES

Increasing your activity helps you lose weight in more ways than you might think. In addition to burning calories, exercise can help you lose weight "in all the right places." Including cardio exercise, like running, biking, or swimming, can increase the number of inches you lose around your waist (a.k.a. belly fat).

Resistance training, such as weight lifting or body weight exercises like push-ups, are important because they help build and preserve muscle mass, which burns more calories (so you can eat more!), but it also helps decrease visceral fat. Visceral fat is the type of fat that surrounds your organs and increases your risk for chronic illnesses. Meal prepping frees up some of your time, so you can begin to incorporate more exercise in your day. You should aim for 150 minutes of moderate exercise per week or 75 minutes of vigorous activity per week.

GENETICS AND PREDISPOSITIONS

Your genetics account for 20 percent of your results, so that means the other 80 percent is in your control. Think of it this way: genetics load the gun and lifestyle pulls the trigger. Unfortunately, you can't change what diseases you may be at risk for, but you can change your lifestyle to help prevent them. Because 80 percent of your risk is in your control, I'd say those are pretty good odds!

THE CLASSIC
1 CARB, 1 PROTEIN, 1 VEGGIE MEAL PREP

Many meal prep fans opt to separately prep one carbohydrate, one protein, and one veggie per meal. This type of meal prep is often preferred because it's easy to batch cook for the whole week. In addition, you can easily follow the "plate method" when determining how much of what to eat. Our recipes in part 3 (see page 111) of this book make it simple to utilize this type of meal prep.

| CARB |
| PROTEIN |
| VEGGIE |

HEALTHY DIETARY PRINCIPLES

The Mediterranean diet and the DASH diet (Dietary Approaches to Stop Hypertension) are two of the most well researched and medically respected eating patterns. Year after year they jostle for the top spot on the list of *U.S. News and World Report*'s Best Diets ranking. Both of these diets can aid weight loss and lower health risks, and that is why this book's recipes are modeled after them.

The Mediterranean diet is based on traditional eating patterns in regions such as Greece and Italy in the 1960s. This diet, really more of a lifestyle, has been shown to aid in weight loss as well as prevent conditions such as heart attack, stroke, and type 2 diabetes. It's a diet that is full of fresh, wonderful flavors and encourages its followers to engage in fun, relaxing activities and social time.

The DASH diet is similar to the Mediterranean diet but strictly reduces salt, sugar, and alcohol intake. It was developed specifically to help people with cardiovascular health issues like hypertension, but has also been shown to be helpful in managing conditions such as type 2 diabetes. Like the Mediterranean diet, it's easy to enjoy a wide variety of delicious foods when following the DASH diet although learning to cook with less sodium can sometimes be intimidating.

Both diets emphasize plant-based meals, heart-healthy fats, low-fat dairy, and lean proteins such as poultry and fish. Furthermore, because these eating patterns are far less restrictive than many other popular "diets," many of my clients find it is easier to create a lasting lifestyle change.

KEEP IT CLEAN AND EASY

Following these general eating patterns is easy when you break it down to the basics. Here are the main components of the "diet" we will be using in this book:

- Select lean meats and fish several times a week and serve red meats sparingly.

- Eat plenty of vegetables with every meal, including those of many different colors.

- Use heart-healthy oils such as avocado oil, olive oil, and canola oil for cooking.

- Serve low-fat dairy products like yogurt and cheese.

- Avoid sugary and processed foods.

- Drink plenty of water.

SPECIAL HEALTH CONSIDERATIONS

Modifications for swaps or substitutions will be provided where possible in case you have gluten or dairy sensitivities, allergies, or intolerances. The meal plans and recipes contain moderate carbohydrate levels, but feel free to modify portion sizes if you need less due to conditions such as insulin resistance. Remember to discuss any health concerns with your doctor before making any dietary change.

ABOUT THE RECIPES

As already mentioned, the recipes in this book contain a delicious mix of the Mediterranean and DASH healthy eating principles, which are as tasty as they are nourishing. All recipes yield multiple servings and are easy to store and reheat well for meal prep. Each recipe will include labels such as dairy-free, DASH, gluten-free, Mediterranean, soy-free, vegetarian, or vegan where applicable.

MAKING SPACE IN YOUR LIFE TO PRIORITIZE YOU

Congratulations on choosing to commit to your health and prioritize healthy eating. It's not easy, but the reward is tenfold. I've always loved this quote:

Those who think they have no time for healthy eating will sooner or later have to find time for illness.

—Edward Stanley

Remember, your commitment to healthy eating is an investment in yourself. To stay consistent, I suggest blocking off times on your calendar to grocery shop and meal prep. Keep those times blocked off like any other appointment you can't miss. If something comes up, make sure to reschedule those times. You've got this.

CUSTOMIZING FOR CALORIES

Calories, as well as other nutrition information, will be included with the recipes. Meals in this book will range between 400 to 600 calories per meal. Remember what we learned about calories earlier: Less is not always better. It would be best if you ate more than your resting metabolic rate and fewer than your total daily expenditure to lose weight.

To calculate your resting metabolic rate (RMR):

Mifflin-St Jeor Equation (calories/day):

Male: $9.99 \times$ weight (kg) $+ 6.25 \times$ height (cm) $- 4.92 \times$ age $+ 5$

Female: $9.99 \times$ weight (kg) $+ 6.25 \times$ height (cm) $- 4.92 \times$ age $- 161$

To calculate your total daily expenditure: RMR $\times$ 1.2 + calories burned in exercise.

MODIFYING CALORIES FOR YOUR UNIQUE NEEDS

Depending on your body's daily needs, you may need to double portion sizes or add snacks to the meal preps included in this book. Some factors that may require you to eat more calories than the portions outlined here include if you are:

- Currently breastfeeding
- Taller than average
- Very active
- A man (men tend to have higher RMRs because they are generally taller and have more muscle mass)

Empower Yourself with Meal Prep

Meal prepping is like the golden ticket to the land of consistency and results. The best part is, the more you practice meal prepping, the faster and more efficient you'll get. Meal prepping also decreases your stress because you'll have healthy meals waiting for you no matter how your week goes.

CONTROL WHAT YOU EAT

Meal prepping puts you in control of what you will eat during the week. Research shows that willpower is like a muscle that can only stand under tension for so long. The more temptations you are exposed to, the harder it is to turn them down. Meal prep helps you control what you eat by exposing you to fewer temptations. With your pre-prepped meals, you are always in control of what you eat, how much you eat, and when you eat.

STOP THE BINGE AND HUNGER CYCLE

Skipping meals often leads to bingeing at the next meal out of extreme hunger. Meal prepping healthy meals stops the hunger and binge cycle because you have meals already prepared and easily available. Research does not show a particular benefit of three meals versus six meals a day, so do what makes sense with your lifestyle and what feels best. Just make sure you eat at least three times a day and at regular intervals.

Breakfast is the most important meal of the day, but it needs to be high in protein. Protein for breakfast reduces cravings and calorie consumption throughout the day. If you aren't hungry for breakfast, try moving dinnertime 30 minutes earlier each night until you are hungry when you wake in the morning.

BREAK FREE OF THE KITCHEN

Meal prepping allows you to cook and clean all at once, and this cuts down the overall time you spend in the kitchen. For instance, you can use the same cutting board to cut and prepare all the vegetables for all the recipes you will make that week. That means you only have to wash that cutting board once. Without meal prepping, you might wash that same cutting board five or more times. You'll save so much time meal prepping you'll be able to break free of the kitchen. Plus, the more you meal prep, the faster and more efficient you'll become, providing valuable hours for you to do the things you love.

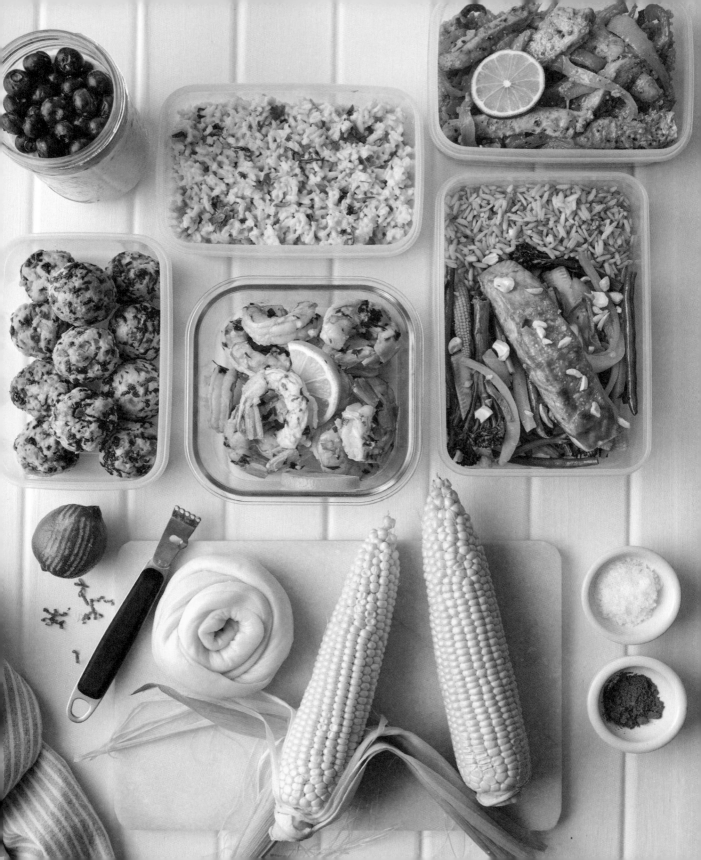

CHAPTER TWO

How to Meal Prep for Weight Loss

We've already determined meal prep is a powerful tool to facilitate weight loss, and now it's time to prepare. This chapter is the "how-to" chapter. I'll walk you through preparation so you have everything you need. We will also discuss the practicality of meal prep, including food safety and food storage options.

Step-by-Step Weight Loss

With a good meal prep plan, weight loss can be as simple as 1-2-3. You are developing a new skill set that you can never unlearn. By learning all about meal prep and following the steps outlined in this book you will be able to lose weight and keep it off.

SET YOUR TARGET

First, it's a good idea to set your goal for what you want to achieve by meal prepping. I love the acronym S.M.A.R.T. for setting goals. It stands for Specific, Measurable, Attainable, Realistic, and Timely. Using this acronym creates accountability for your goals.

For example, let's turn the generic goal of "weight loss" into a S.M.A.R.T. goal. You might say your goal is **to lose 8 pounds by June 1st by meal prepping once a week on Sundays at 10 a.m.**

Take a minute to write down your own S.M.A.R.T goal answering these questions:

- How much weight do you want to lose?

- When will you achieve this goal?

- How often will you meal prep?

- When will you meal prep?

WHAT TO EAT?

As mentioned before, we will follow the plate method for creating nutritional balance in our meals. Balanced meals lead to better energy levels, fewer cravings, and sustainable weight loss. This section covers what to fill your meal prep container with to help you lose weight and keep it off—permanently.

Protein stimulates metabolism, balances blood sugar, builds lean tissue, and supports immune function. Include a protein source at every meal, including egg whites, high-protein dairy products (cottage cheese and Greek yogurt), poultry, fish, shellfish, lean beef cuts (like 96 percent lean ground beef), lean pork cuts (like boneless pork chops), lentils, tofu, or edamame.

Produce is abundant in life-sustaining and disease-fighting antioxidants, vitamins, minerals, and phytochemicals. These nutrients are best absorbed from food versus taken as supplements. Produce also provides fiber, which helps keep you fuller longer. Most fiber comes from non-starchy vegetables, which include but are not limited to:

- Artichokes
- Asparagus
- Bean sprouts
- Bell peppers
- Broccoli
- Brussels sprouts
- Cabbage
- Cauliflower
- Celery
- Cucumbers
- Eggplants

- Mushrooms
- Onions
- Peppers
- Salad greens
- Spinach
- Squash (all types: spaghetti, yellow, acorn, delicata, etc.)
- Sweet mini peppers
- Tomatoes
- Turnips
- Zucchini

When it comes to starch and weight loss, both quality and quantity matter. High-quality carbohydrates are those in the least processed form, which have higher levels of filling protein and fiber. Examples include, but are not limited to:

- Barley
- Beans (except lentils and edamame)
- Brown rice
- Corn
- Couscous
- Farro
- Oats

- Peas
- Plantains
- Potatoes
- Quinoa
- Sweet potatoes
- Whole fruit (not fruit juice)
- Whole wheat

Don't fear fat. It is essential to metabolism and function. Your brain is 60 percent fat; hormones are made from fat; and every cell in your body is surrounded by fat. Opt for several servings per day of the following foods:

- Avocados
- Egg yolks
- Fatty fish like salmon and tuna
- Olives
- Organic grass-fed dairy products
- Nuts including peanuts, and seeds

I also recommend cooking with unrefined cold-pressed avocado oil and using olive oil for colder items like salad dressings.

HOW MUCH TO EAT?

Your overall caloric needs are unique to you, but if you focus on setting up your portions using these guidelines you'll be off to a good start in meeting them. Recipes in the meal plans follow this setup so you'll gain some practice cooking meals that follow this portion guide.

Carbohydrates: Some carbohydrates break down into sugar in the body and some carbohydrates are indigestible (fiber), passing through the GI system untouched. Both non-starchy vegetables and starchy vegetables provide carbohydrates. Modify this amount as needed, aiming for about 40 percent of your calories coming from carbohydrates, but not exceeding 45-ish grams per meal. If you are very active (for example, training for a marathon) you may need to increase this amount, up to 65 percent, exceeding the 45 grams per meal guideline. Otherwise, stick with 40 percent.

Aim to get a minimum of 25 grams and 40 grams of fiber, for women and men respectively. Please don't worry about net carbs (total carbs minus fiber); just get in your minimum fiber for the day. That said, there are some recipes in this book that exceed 45 grams of carbs per recipe but not 45 grams of net carbs. Try not to get too caught up or obsessed with the numbers; the ultimate goal is to create balance in each meal and throughout the day.

Non-starchy veggies: Your fists are proportionate to your body, so they are a great way to eyeball portion sizes. Aim for two fistfuls of vegetables at each meal, for at least two meals a day.

Starch: About ½ cup, or 30 to 45 grams, per meal is appropriate for most people trying to lose weight.

Protein: One palm-size (4- to 6-ounce) portion should equal 20 to 30 grams of protein. Most women should get one portion and men should get two portions at each meal.

Healthy fat: Aim for 1 to 2 tablespoons per meal or snack. Fat is calorie dense, so you do need to watch your portions, but it's also filling so don't skip it. Just make sure there is a little healthy fat in the meal either added at the end or during the cooking process.

Drinks: Water, black tea, coffee, infused fruit water, and sparkling water are great options. For weight loss, weight maintenance, and general health, avoid high-sugar beverages such as soda, juice, sports drinks, and other drinks with added sugars.

MAKE YOUR PLAN

To create a meal prep plan, you must first create a quick meal plan.

1. Look in your cabinets and freezer and make a list of things you need to use up.

2. Use the ingredients to plan recipes into your week.

3. Make a list of the recipes you want to prep ahead of time.

4. Make a list of ingredients you don't have that you need to make the recipes you selected.

What I Have	Recipes to Make	What I Need

SELECTING RECIPES

Almost any recipe can be meal-prep friendly, but there are a few things to keep in mind when selecting recipes to make, such as:

- Does it contain healthy ingredients (free of processed foods)?

- Does it follow the plate method, or can it be modified to follow this method?

- Will the food be easy to store?

- Will the food reheat well? Example: The air fryer craze is fun, but the food doesn't reheat nearly as crispy and tasty as you'd like.

GATHER WHAT YOU NEED

Having some basic kitchen gear will allow you to begin meal prepping with ease. This section outlines the equipment and tools needed for meal prep, and offers some tips to keep grocery costs down.

HELPFUL TOOLS AND EQUIPMENT

Kitchen Equipment

Not a lot is required to begin meal prepping. These kitchen basics will get you started:

- 8-by-8-inch casserole dish

- 9-by-13-inch casserole dish

- Aluminum foil, heavy-duty

- Baking sheets (2)

- Large nonstick skillet with lid

- Muffin tin with silicone liners or silicone muffin tin

- Oven

- Oven-safe skillet

- Slow cooker

- Stovetop

Meal Prep Equipment

- Airtight storage containers

- Divided airtight storage containers

- Insulated lunch bag for transporting food

- Mason jars and lids

SHOPPING IN BULK

Shopping in bulk is a great way to save money and always be prepared for meal prepping. Freeze unused portions for use in future meal preps. Food items that are great to purchase in bulk are:

- Beans
- Cooking oils
- Fish
- Grains (oats, quinoa, etc.)

- Nuts
- Poultry
- Seeds
- Shellfish

Note: Bulk bins are not suitable for those with food allergies as foods can easily become cross-contaminated with potential allergens.

Throughout the book, I use avocado oil for cooking. Unrefined cold-pressed avocado oil is very stable at high temperatures and has similar health benefits to olive oil. When purchased in bulk, the price point is comparable to olive oil. However, you can substitute canola oil or olive oil for avocado oil in any recipe in this book.

Chickpea flour is a high-protein flour utilized in a few recipes in this book. Whole-wheat flour can be used instead of chickpea flour but, when purchased in bulk, chickpea flour can be very affordable.

For weight loss, my preferred baking flour is almond flour because its fat and protein content is more satiating. You cannot substitute any other flour for almond flour because it is a high-fat, high-protein flour. Almond flour can be purchased in bulk to save money.

Other Ways to Keep Costs Down:

- Avoid purchasing items in bulk that might go bad and can't be frozen, such as dairy.
- Buy beans canned.
- Cook meatless meals one night per week.
- Eat from the pantry (use what you have).

- Freeze unused fruit for smoothies.
- Limit more expensive organic purchases to the EWG Dirty Dozen™ list (see page 169).
- Shop sales and use coupons.
- Shop seasonal produce.

EXECUTE EFFICIENTLY

The goal of meal prepping is to learn to be as efficient as possible, so you spend the least amount of time in the kitchen, but make the most of it for your healthy eating goals. You will naturally get faster at meal prep the more practice you have. This section provides time-saving tips to get you started.

PLANNING THE COOK SESSION

In general, work from the most time-consuming item to the least. For example:

1. Slow cooker recipes should be started first.

2. Recipes with long cooking times go in the oven next.

3. Sheet pan recipes with shorter cooking times follow.

4. Hands-on stovetop recipes follow.

5. No-bake recipes are completed last.

Decide whether you will do one or two preps per week, then split up the meals accordingly. Depending on the selected recipes and your schedule in a given week, you may choose to do one prep some weeks and two preps per week at other times.

EFFORT-SAVING TIPS AND TRICKS

1. Cook items in bulk that can be used for various meals, such as brown rice, quinoa, or shredded chicken, and freeze the remaining portion for another week.

2. You don't have to cook every single meal for the whole week. Cook ingredients that take time but are components of your selected recipes, like grains, for use in recipes later in the week.

3. If budget allows, purchase already cut and washed produce. You can also use frozen foods to save time on prep work.

4. Repeat meals. Make sure you provide variety from week to week but, during the week, repeat meals as often as possible to save time in the kitchen.

5. Use the same ingredients in multiple recipes.

PORTION AND STORE

Now that you've cooked your meal, you need to know how much to eat and how to store the remaining food in meal-prepped portions.

WHAT'S THE RIGHT PORTION SIZE?

Follow the plate method to determine portions for protein, carbs, and veggies. For mixed entrées, eyeball it (using your palm and fist as a size guide, see pages 16–17) or use the nutrition facts with the recipe as your guideline. If you use the nutrition facts, you are aiming for 400 to 600 calories, 25 grams of protein for females and 35 grams for males, about 15 grams of fat for females and up to 32 grams for males, and 30 to 45 grams of carbs (dependent on activity levels and prior health conditions) per meal.

Adjust the portion sizes of a recipe to get as close to that as possible without driving yourself crazy. If using the plate method, you'll be pretty close without counting anything. In general, a good dose of protein, a moderate amount of carbs, and a ton of veggies are what you want on your plate (or in your meal prep container).

FRIDGE VERSUS FREEZER

First, check the expiration of your ingredients as you go. If you use yogurt about to expire tomorrow in a recipe today, then that recipe that might normally be good for 3 days may be bad tomorrow. Once food has been cooked, it's generally considered edible for 3 to 5 days. If you think you won't use it in that time, throw it in the freezer to eat later. However, I regularly meal prep for up to 6 days and find that many foods do just fine in the refrigerator for that amount of time.

The freezer has the advantage of keeping foods safe for 3 to 6 months, making it a good alternative to extend the shelf life of your meal-prepped foods. A few tips for freezer success are:

- Freeze meals in individual portions so you can reheat just one meal at a time.

- Store food in airtight containers, wrapped with plastic wrap to protect further against freezer burn.

- Clearly label the food and the date you froze it.

- Liquids expand when they freeze, so leave room in the container for this. In general, leave at least 40 percent of the container empty for expansion.

Prepared food should sit out for no more than 2 hours at room temperature; if it does, it needs to be consumed within 4 hours, or tossed. Once the food is cooked, it should be reheated to a temperature of 165°F before serving it again (regardless of whether you froze it or not). In most cases, you don't need to use a thermometer; just cook your food until it's steaming. However, certain immune-compromised populations, such as the elderly, children, and pregnant women, may want to use a thermometer to ensure their food is reheated to 165°F.

Leftover and Reheating Guide

Successful meal prepping relies on storing leftovers safely and reheating food properly, so it still tastes good. This section offers useful tips and tricks on repurposing leftovers and creating the best possible experience when reheating food.

REPURPOSING LEFTOVERS

There are two types of leftovers: entire recipes and individual ingredients for meals.

If you have an entire entrée or side dish "leftover" you can:

- Freeze unused portions of food to eat later or for use in a future recipe.

- If there isn't enough left over to call it a full meal, use what you have as a side dish to your next meal.

- Use side dishes as ingredients in a meal. Leftover cubed sweet potato? Add it to an egg scramble or other meal.

- Eat dinner for breakfast or breakfast for dinner. Don't be tied to conventional norms of which foods should be eaten when. If you have a leftover stack of meal-prepped pancakes, eat those bad boys for dinner—no one is stopping you but you. The opposite is true as well if you have a leftover chicken, eat it for breakfast.

- When it comes to repurposing leftovers, start thinking of them as ingredients, not leftovers. You might be able to make an entirely new meal from the leftovers of a different meal.

- Have a leftover night where you eat the last little bits of whatever is left, clearing out the fridge.

The second type of leftover is leftover ingredients. If you are following the plans and recipes in this book, this may be more of a concern than entire leftover meals. For example, a recipe might call for half a can of coconut milk. What do you do with the other half?

- Utilize the freezer when possible. Transfer the food to a freezer-safe container, mark the item, amount left, and the date. Freezing food is an excellent option for things like leftover jarred sauces or canned liquids.

- Fruit can be frozen for smoothies.

- Wilting salad greens can be sautéed and added to eggs, ground meat, or even "hidden" in smoothies.

- Leftover coconut milk or other milk can be frozen in ice cubes for use in smoothies.

- Leftover veggies can be thrown into an "everything but the kitchen sink" salad or soup.

TASTY REHEATED FOOD

For best results when reheating foods, the general rule of thumb is to "reheat" the food in the mode in which it was cooked. However, the recipes in this book consider that you likely do not want to dirty cookware and may not be at home when you are eating meals, so all meals can be reheated in the microwave. That said, some of the following tips may help improve the quality of your reheated meals in the microwave.

1. For red meat and chicken, add a little water (no more than 1 tablespoon) to help your meal retain moisture when microwaving.

2. For fish, be sure to cover the container when reheating. Fish has a habit of "popping" and exploding all over the microwave. The best way to avoid this is

to cover it and use increasing heat levels. For example, start with low power for 20 seconds, then medium power for 20 seconds, then medium-high power for 1 minute, and so on.

3. When reheating baked, fried, and roasted food, the best method to use is the oven to reheat it. If you have access to a convection oven and can cover the tray with aluminum foil (to avoid cleanup), this is the best option. If you need to use a microwave to do the reheating, place a glass of water in it along with the food while you reheat it to help decrease the "sogginess" factor.

4. Sautéed, stir-fried, and steamed food generally does well with microwave reheating. Make sure to stir it halfway through the cooking time to facilitate even heating. You may also want to sprinkle the food with a little water to prevent it from drying out.

5. Defrosting frozen food in the refrigerator overnight is the ideal method of thawing it. If that isn't possible, use either the defrost setting or half power when thawing food in the microwave.

No access to a microwave? You can get a portable oven food reheater for a decent price. Look online for deals on these handy gadgets that can make meal prepping much easier if you need to reheat at the office or on the go.

About the Meal Plans and Recipes

In part 2, I've put together eight separate meal plans with step-by-step instructions for meal prep, grocery lists, and recipes. If you work your way through the meal preps from chapter 3 through 6, you'll start off with three recipes per week and work your way up to six. As you practice, you'll get more efficient with both technique and time, so that by the time you get to the six-recipe meal preps, you'll be much quicker in your work than when you started with the three-recipe prep.

In part 3, I've provided batch-friendly recipes. Once you've completed the meal prep plans and are ready to put together your own meal plan, the recipes in this section will help you be most efficient with your time. Selected to make it easy to throw together one protein, one veggie, and one carb for each meal, the recipes can be scaled up or down easily for servings depending on what you need. All recipes include calorie customization tips and instructions for freezing.

STEAMED VEGETABLES

Don't forget, lightly steaming vegetables is a delicious and easy option as well. Follow the chart to steam these common vegetables. Keep in mind that because you will also be reheating them (leading to more cooking), steam many of these veggies lightly!

APPROXIMATE STEAMING TIMES FOR VEGETABLES:

Asparagus spears	7 to 13 minutes
Broccoli florets	8 to 12 minutes
Brussels sprouts	8 to 10 minutes
Carrots	7 to 10 minutes
Cauliflower florets	5 to 10 minutes
Eggplant	7 to 9 minutes
Green beans	3 to 5 minutes
Sugar snap peas	6 to 7 minutes

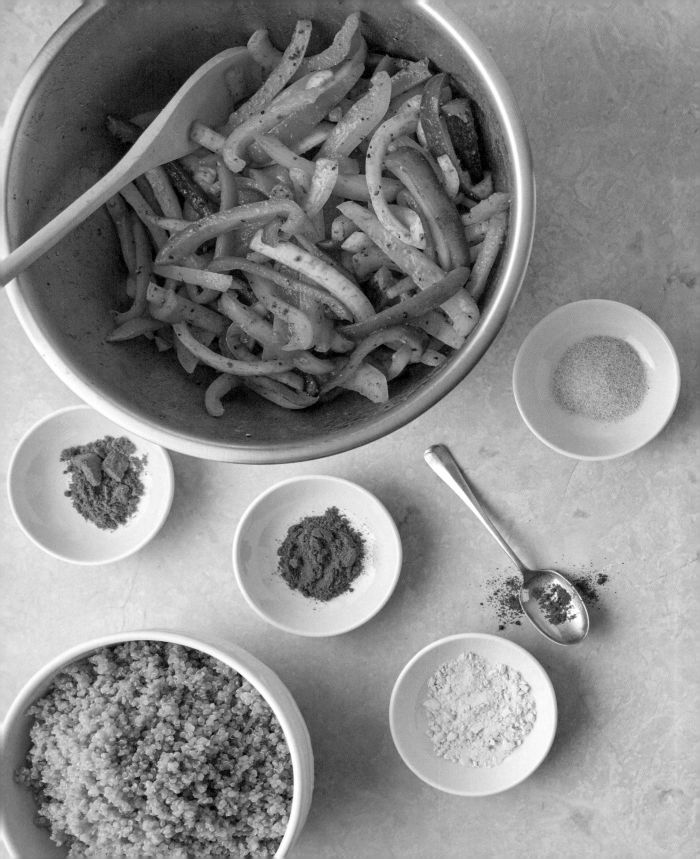

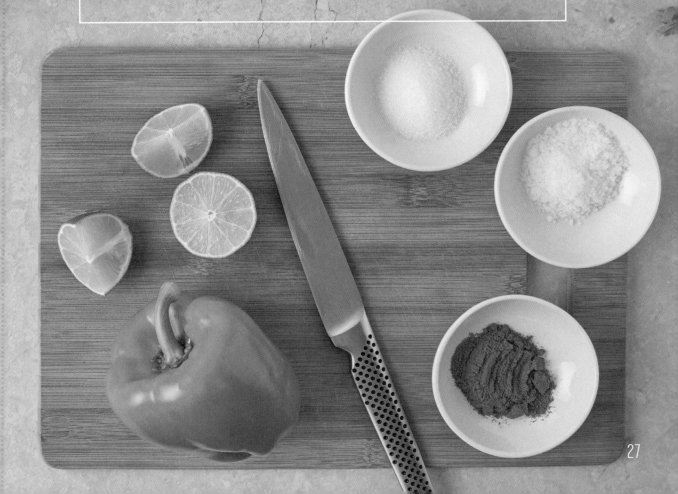
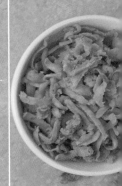

PART TWO

WEIGHT LOSS
Meal Prep Plans with
RECIPES

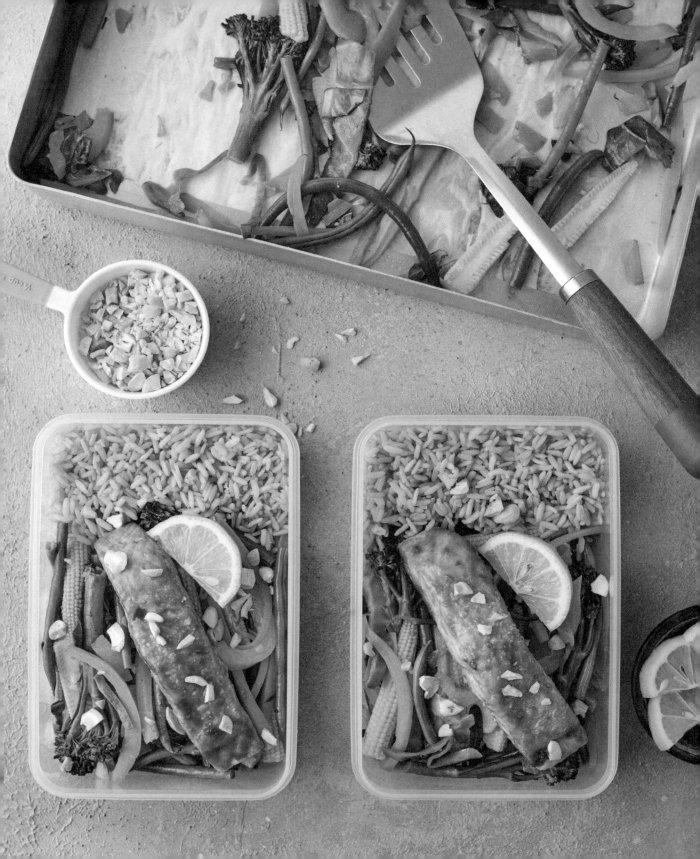

CHAPTER THREE

Basic Three-Recipe Meal Preps

Five-Day Breakfast and Lunch Meal Prep Plan 30

One-Pan Crispy Chicken Thighs with
Roasted Red Potatoes and Green Beans 32

Make-Ahead Fruit and Yogurt Parfaits 34

Customizable Finger Foods Lunch 35

Five-Day Prep Lunch and Dinner Meal Plan 36

Slow Cooker Spaghetti Squash Turkey Bolognese 38

Chopped Rainbow Mediterranean Salad 40

Sheet Pan Sweet and Spicy Salmon with Veggies 42

《 Sheet Pan Sweet and Spicy Salmon with Veggies (page 42)

Five-Day Breakfast and Lunch Meal Prep Plan

Breakfast and lunch are a great way to start meal prepping because you are most likely to skip these meals when life gets busy. Research consistently shows that breakfast eaters weigh less and have fewer health concerns, so it's essential to eat a substantial breakfast that includes protein every single day. If you're someone who isn't typically hungry for breakfast, move your dinnertime 30 minutes earlier each night until you wake hungry.

This plan was created to show you that meal prepping can be easy and doesn't have to require hours in the kitchen. You only have to "cook" one of these recipes and the rest are put together without ever turning on the stove.

SHOPPING LIST

PANTRY
- Almond butter
- Almonds, slivered
- Black pepper, freshly ground
- Italian seasoning, salt-free
- Nonstick cooking spray
- Oil, avocado
- Sea salt
- Stevia drops, vanilla

CANNED, BOTTLED, PACKAGED, AND PREPARED
- Hummus (¾ cup)
- Gluten-free whole-grain crackers (3 servings)

FRUITS, VEGETABLES, FRESH HERBS, AND SPICES
- Carrots, baby (3 cups)
- Green beans (12 ounces)
- Onion, sweet (1)
- Peppers, sweet mini (3 cups)
- Red potatoes (8 ounces)

PROTEIN
- Chicken thighs, bone-in (1½ pounds)
- Deli turkey (12 ounces)

DAIRY
- Cheese, Havarti (3 ounces)
- Yogurt, plain nonfat Greek (5 cups)

FROZEN
- Blueberries (2½ cups)
- Strawberries (2½ cups)

EQUIPMENT LIST
- Baking sheet
- Chef's knife
- Cutting board
- Food thermometer
- Measuring cups and spoons
- Mixing bowls
- Parchment paper
- Pint-size Mason jars
- Resealable quart-size plastic bags
- Storage containers

	Breakfast	**Lunch**
DAY 1	Make-Ahead Fruit and Yogurt Parfaits (page 34)	One-Pan Crispy Chicken Thighs with Roasted Red Potatoes and Green Beans (page 32)
DAY 2	Make-Ahead Fruit and Yogurt Parfaits (page 34)	One-Pan Crispy Chicken Thighs with Roasted Red Potatoes and Green Beans (page 32)
DAY 3	Make-Ahead Fruit and Yogurt Parfaits (page 34)	Customizable Finger Foods Lunch (page 35)
DAY 4	Make-Ahead Fruit and Yogurt Parfaits (page 34)	Customizable Finger Foods Lunch (page 35)
DAY 5	Make-Ahead Fruit and Yogurt Parfaits (page 34)	Customizable Finger Foods Lunch (page 35)

STEP-BY-STEP GUIDE

1. Preheat the oven to 425°F.

2. Start by making the **One-Pan Crispy Chicken Thighs with Roasted Red Potatoes and Green Beans** (page 32) and place it in the oven to bake.

3. While the chicken cooks, prepare the **Make-Ahead Fruit and Yogurt Parfaits** (page 34) and refrigerate them.

4. Prepare the **Customizable Finger Foods Lunch** (page 35) and refrigerate.

5. When the chicken thighs are cooked through, portion the thighs, potatoes, and green beans into airtight storage containers, cool, seal, and refrigerate.

One-Pan Crispy Chicken Thighs *with* Roasted Red Potatoes *and* Green Beans

PREP TIME: 15 minutes | COOK TIME: 40 minutes

This easy sheet pan meal yields tender succulent chicken thighs and savory roasted veggies. Though I use potatoes and green beans in this recipe, you can improvise other vegetables you have on hand to make endless combinations of this simple dish.

12 ounces green beans, trimmed

8 ounces red potatoes, halved

½ sweet onion, sliced

1 tablespoon avocado oil

2 teaspoons salt-free Italian seasoning, divided

½ teaspoon sea salt, divided

½ teaspoon freshly ground black pepper, divided

1½ pounds bone-in chicken thighs

Nonstick cooking spray

DAIRY-FREE • GLUTEN-FREE • MEDITERRANEAN • SOY-FREE

1. Preheat the oven to 425°F and line a baking sheet with parchment paper or aluminum foil.

2. On the baking sheet, spread the green beans, potatoes, and onion evenly across three-quarters of the sheet. Pour the avocado oil over the veggies. Sprinkle with 1 teaspoon Italian seasoning, ¼ teaspoon of salt, and ¼ teaspoon of pepper. Toss to coat.

3. Season the chicken thighs with the remaining 1 teaspoon of Italian seasoning, ¼ teaspoon of salt, and ¼ teaspoon of pepper. Coat the empty portion of the sheet, where the chicken will go, with cooking spray and place the chicken thighs, skin-side up, on the prepared area.

4. Bake for 30 minutes until the chicken reaches an internal temperature of 165°F and the veggies are fork-tender.

5. If desired, for added crispness, adjust the oven to broil. Broil for 3 to 7 minutes until the chicken is browned.

NEED MORE CALORIES? Double the portion of chicken and vegetables for more protein and carbs. You may need to use two sheet pans, but you can cook a double batch at once. Switch the pans to the opposite rack and turn them front to back halfway through the cooking time and broil each separately.

STORAGE TIP: Freeze the meal in individual portions. Thaw in the refrigerator overnight and reheat to 165°F.

INGREDIENT TIP: Want a different flavor profile? Swap Italian seasoning for poultry seasoning or any other seasoning blend you like.

Although this recipe is indicated as gluten-free, if this is a concern for you, check the ingredient packaging to ensure all foods were processed in a completely gluten-free facility.

Per Serving (½ recipe): Calories: 516; Fat: 26g; Carbohydrates: 37g; Fiber: 7g; Protein: 35g; Sodium: 736mg

Make-Ahead Fruit *and* Yogurt Parfaits

PREP TIME: 15 minutes

These make-ahead fruit and yogurt parfaits are creamy, delicious, and amazingly simple to put together. Almond butter adds a rich flavor to the yogurt and the berries and almonds add texture and bursts of sweetness to each bite.

5 cups plain nonfat Greek yogurt

5 tablespoons almond butter

15 drops vanilla stevia

2½ cups frozen blueberries

2½ cups frozen strawberries

5 tablespoons slivered almonds

DASH • GLUTEN-FREE • SOY-FREE • VEGETARIAN

1.   In a large bowl, stir together the yogurt, almond butter, and stevia until well combined.

2.   In each of the 5 pint-size Mason jars, in the following order, layer ½ cup of blueberries, ½ cup of yogurt mixture, ½ cup of strawberries, and top with ½ cup of the yogurt mixture.

3.   Top each parfait with 1 tablespoon of slivered almonds. Close the lids tightly and refrigerate.

NEED MORE CALORIES? Double the portions of all the ingredients (use larger Mason jars or containers) or double the yogurt mixture by following the same layering process and using 1 cup of yogurt per layer.

STORAGE TIP: Keep refrigerated for up to 5 days. Do not freeze.

INGREDIENT TIP: Fresh berries can be substituted for frozen if available.

Although this recipe is indicated as gluten-free, if this is a concern for you, check the ingredient packaging to ensure all foods were processed in a completely gluten-free facility.

Per Serving (1 parfait): Calories: 386; Fat: 18g; Carbohydrates: 33g; Fiber: 6g; Protein: 28g; Sodium: 145mg

Customizable Finger Foods Lunch

PREP TIME: 15 minutes

A finger food lunch is the ultimate easy meal prep. All you have to do is decide which combination of protein, veggie, fat, and carb you want and place the items in the box. If you have divided storage containers, this is the perfect place to use them.

12 ounces deli turkey meat

3 Havarti cheese slices, halved

3 cups baby carrots

3 cups sweet mini peppers

¾ cup hummus

3 servings whole-grain crackers

SOY-FREE

1. Roll 2 pieces of turkey around each half slice of Havarti cheese. Into each of 3 storage containers, place 2 roll-ups, 1 cup carrots, and 1 cup mini peppers.

2. Place ¼ cup of hummus into each of 3 small storage containers and divide the crackers among 3 resealable plastic bags and seal.

> **NEED MORE CALORIES?** You may need to double the portions of turkey and cheese to get enough calories, protein, and fat. To decrease the calories, reduce the hummus to 2 tablespoons per serving or omit it entirely.

STORAGE TIP: This recipe is not freezer friendly. Keep refrigerated and enjoy within 3 days.

INGREDIENT TIP: Swap deli chicken or ham for the turkey. Swap guacamole or nut butter for hummus and cheese. (This substitution will also make this meal dairy-free.) Other finger food veggies such as sugar snap peas, cherry tomatoes, or mini cucumbers can be used. Swap 1 cup fruit or a piece of dark chocolate for your carb. (This substitution will also make this meal gluten-free.)

Per Serving (1 lunch): Calories: 518; Fat: 24g; Carbohydrates: 43g; Fiber: 10g; Protein: 34g; Sodium: 1,805mg

Five-Day Prep Lunch and Dinner Meal Plan

Now that you've got one meal prep done, it's time to take things up a notch. This meal plan will teach you how to be super efficient with your prep work. The plan utilizes three different preparation methods: slow cooking, roasting, and mixing cold ingredients—all at one time. You'll work from the recipe that takes the most time to the one that takes the least during your prep, so you'll be as efficient as possible.

SHOPPING LIST

PANTRY
- Black pepper, freshly ground
- Cashews
- Cornstarch
- Garlic sea salt
- Ginger, ground
- Honey
- Nonstick cooking spray
- Oil, avocado
- Oil, olive, extra-virgin
- Oil, sesame
- Soy sauce, low-sodium
- Sriracha

CANNED, BOTTLED, PACKAGED, AND PREPARED
- Bolognese sauce (1 [24-ounce] jar)
- Chickpeas (1 [15-ounce] can)

FRUITS, VEGETABLES, FRESH HERBS, AND SPICES
- Bell pepper, orange (1)
- Bell pepper, red (1)
- Bell pepper, yellow (1)
- Cucumbers (3)
- Garlic (1 head)
- Lemon (1)
- Mushrooms (6 ounces [2 cups chopped])
- Onion, yellow (1)
- Parsley (1 bunch)
- Squash, spaghetti, very large (1)
- Stir-fry vegetables (1 [24-ounce] package)
- Tomatoes, cherry (3 cups)

PROTEIN
- Chicken breast, boneless, skinless (20 ounces)
- Salmon fillets (1 pound)
- Turkey sausage, Italian (1 pound)

DAIRY
- Cheese, feta (2 ounces [⅓ cup])
- Cheese, shredded mozzarella (3 ounces [¾ cup])

EQUIPMENT LIST
- Airtight storage containers
- Aluminum foil
- Baking sheets
- Chef's knife
- Cutting board
- Food thermometer
- Large skillet
- Measuring cups and spoons
- Mixing bowls
- Parchment paper
- Resealable quart-size plastic bags
- Slow cooker

	Lunch	Dinner
DAY 1	Chopped Rainbow Mediterranean Salad (page 40)	Sheet Pan Sweet and Spicy Salmon with Veggies (page 42)
DAY 2	Chopped Rainbow Mediterranean Salad (page 40)	Sheet Pan Sweet and Spicy Salmon with Veggies (page 42)
DAY 3	Chopped Rainbow Mediterranean Salad (page 40)	Slow Cooker Spaghetti Squash Turkey Bolognese (page 38)
DAY 4	Chopped Rainbow Mediterranean Salad (page 40)	Slow Cooker Spaghetti Squash Turkey Bolognese (page 38)
DAY 5	Chopped Rainbow Mediterranean Salad (page 40)	Slow Cooker Spaghetti Squash Turkey Bolognese (page 38)

STEP-BY-STEP GUIDE

1. Start by prepping the **Slow Cooker Spaghetti Squash Turkey Bolognese** (page 38) through step 3.

2. Preheat the oven to 400°F.

3. Prepare the **Chopped Rainbow Mediterranean Salad** (page 40) through step 4.

4. Prepare the **Sheet Pan Sweet and Spicy Salmon with Veggies** (page 42) through step 3. The salmon and chicken can go into the oven together at the same time.

5. Prepare the sauce for the salmon.

6. Prepare the salad portion of the **Chopped Rainbow Mediterranean Salad**. The salmon will likely be done before you finish preparing the salad. Stop prepping the salad and finish the salmon through the end of the recipe, including portioning it and then returning to preparing your vegetables.

7. Finish and portion the salad.

8. Finish and portion the spaghetti squash recipe.

Slow Cooker Spaghetti Squash Turkey Bolognese

PREP TIME: 15 minutes | COOK TIME: 4 to 6 hours

The slow cooker marinates this classic meaty Bolognese sauce with mushrooms and sweet Italian ground turkey for hours until the aromas of garlic and tomato sauce take over the kitchen. If you are not a fan of mushrooms, substitute zucchini or eggplant in their place.

1 tablespoon avocado oil

1 yellow onion, chopped

1 pound Italian turkey sausage

1 (24-ounce) jar Bolognese sauce

2 cups chopped mushrooms

1 very large spaghetti squash or 2 small spaghetti squashes, halved and seeded

¾ cup shredded mozzarella cheese

3 tablespoons fresh parsley, divided

GLUTEN-FREE • MEDITERRANEAN • SOY-FREE

1.   In a large skillet, heat the avocado oil over medium-high heat. Add the onion and sauté for 3 to 5 minutes until translucent and tender. Add the sausage to the skillet, and cook until it is no longer pink, for about 10 minutes.

2.   In a slow cooker, stir together the Bolognese sauce, sausage and onion, and mushrooms.

3.   Place the spaghetti squash, cut-side down, on top of the sauce.

4.   Cover the slow cooker and cook on high heat for 4 to 6 hours, or on low heat for 6 to 8 hours, until the spaghetti squash is fork-tender.

5. When the spaghetti squash is done, using a fork, shred the squash and remove the strands from the outer shell and divide them among 3 storage containers. Top each with one-third of the sauce, ¼ cup of mozzarella cheese, and 1 tablespoon of parsley.

6. When ready to eat, reheat the spaghetti squash in the microwave.

NEED MORE CALORIES? Double the portion of turkey sausage.

STORAGE TIP: Freeze the meal in individual portions. Thaw in the refrigerator overnight and reheat to 165°F.

INGREDIENT TIP: Although this recipe is indicated as gluten-free, if this is a concern for you, check the ingredient packaging to ensure all foods were processed in a completely gluten-free facility.

Per Serving (⅓ recipe): Calories: 510; Fat: 28g; Carbohydrates: 31g; Fiber: 6g; Protein: 35g; Sodium: 1,365mg

Chopped Rainbow Mediterranean Salad

PREP TIME: 30 minutes | COOK TIME: 40 minutes

Every bite of this salad is crunchy, juicy, and refreshing from the first to the last day you eat it. Plus, it's packed with colorful vegetables that supply anti-inflammatory antioxidants, phytonutrients, vitamins, and minerals.

Nonstick cooking spray

20 ounces boneless, skinless chicken breast

2 teaspoons garlic sea salt, divided

1 teaspoon freshly ground black pepper, divided

3 cucumbers, halved lengthwise, cut into ½-inch half-moons

1 red bell pepper, cut into ½-inch pieces

1 orange bell pepper, cut into ½-inch pieces

1 yellow bell pepper, cut into ½-inch pieces

3 cups cherry tomatoes, halved

1 (15-ounce) can chickpeas, drained and rinsed

⅓ cup feta cheese

2½ tablespoons extra-virgin olive oil

1½ tablespoons freshly squeezed lemon juice

DASH • GLUTEN-FREE • MEDITERRANEAN • SOY-FREE

1. Preheat the oven to 400°F. Line a baking sheet with parchment paper and coat it with cooking spray.

2. Sprinkle the chicken breasts all over with 1 teaspoon of garlic salt and ½ teaspoon of pepper. Place them on the prepared baking sheet and bake for 30 to 40 minutes until its internal temperature reaches 165°F.

3. In a large mixing bowl, toss together the cucumbers, bell peppers, and tomatoes. Add the chickpeas, cheese, olive oil, lemon, the remaining 1 teaspoon of garlic salt, and the remaining ½ teaspoon of pepper and toss well to combine. Divide the salad evenly among 5 storage containers.

4. When the chicken is finished baking, cut it into 1-inch cubes and let cool completely.

5. Portion out the chicken, cover, and refrigerate.

NEED MORE CALORIES? Increase the chicken to 30 ounces and double the amount of feta cheese.

STORAGE TIP: Serve cold. Do not freeze or reheat.

INGREDIENT TIP: Although this recipe is indicated as gluten-free, check the ingredient packaging to ensure all foods were processed in a completely gluten-free facility.

Per Serving (⅕ recipe): Calories: 368; Fat: 14g; Carbohydrates: 31g; Fiber: 7g; Protein: 35g; Sodium: 428mg

Sheet Pan Sweet *and* Spicy Salmon *with* Veggies

PREP TIME: 10 minutes | COOK TIME: 20 minutes

Salmon is loaded with omega-3s and is easy to cook, making it a perfect choice for healthy eating and meal prep. Paired with stir-fry vegetables roasted to perfection then doused with a succulent sweet and spicy glaze, this meal makes a perfect lunch or dinner option. Look for pre-cut vegetables in your grocery's refrigerated produce section to make prep even easier.

---

1 (24-ounce) package stir-fry vegetables

1 tablespoon sesame oil

1 pound salmon fillets

Nonstick cooking spray

⅓ cup low-sodium soy sauce

2 tablespoons Sriracha

2 tablespoons honey

1 teaspoon cornstarch

2 garlic cloves, minced

¼ teaspoon ground ginger

2 tablespoons crushed cashews

DAIRY-FREE • MEDITERRANEAN

---

1. Preheat the oven to 400°F and line two baking sheets with aluminum foil.

2. Spread the stir-fry vegetables on one baking sheet and toss them with the sesame oil to coat. Place the baking sheet on the top or middle rack in the oven.

3. Coat the skin side of the salmon with cooking spray and place the salmon, skin-side down, on the second baking sheet. Place that baking sheet on the bottom rack of the oven.

4. Bake for 20 minutes, or until the salmon is cooked all the way through, flaking easily with a fork, and the vegetables are fork-tender.

5.   While the salmon and vegetables roast, in a small sauce-pan over medium heat, whisk the soy sauce, Sriracha, honey, cornstarch, garlic, and ginger. Cook for 5 to 7 minutes until thickened, stirring occasionally. If the sauce starts to boil, turn down the heat.

6.   When the salmon is done, brush it with the sauce. Toss the vegetables with the remaining sauce and garnish them with the cashews.

7.   Into each of 2 storage containers, place 1 salmon fillet and half the veggies.

STORAGE TIP: Freeze the meal in individual portions. Thaw overnight in the refrigerator and reheat to 165°F in microwave.

INGREDIENT TIP: To make this recipe gluten-free and soy-free, use coconut aminos instead of the soy sauce.

Per Serving (½ recipe): Calories: 490; Fat: 22g; Carbohydrates: 30g; Fiber: 3g; Protein: 39g; Sodium: 1,968mg

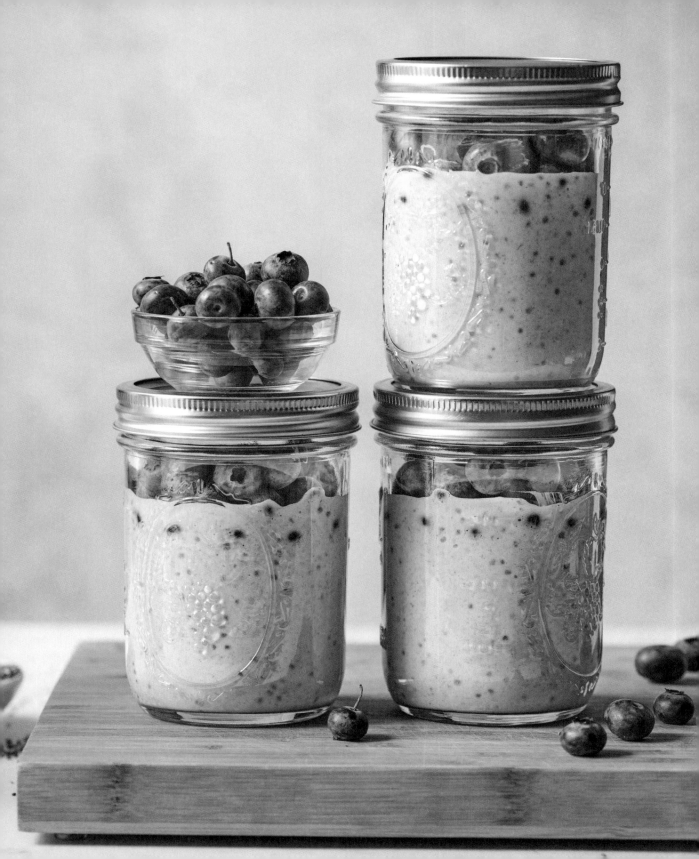

CHAPTER FOUR

Batch-Friendly Four-Recipe Meal Preps

First Quick and Easy Three-Day Meal Prep Plan 46

Italian Marinated Grilled Chicken 48

Garlic and Herb Farro with Lemon-Pepper Broccoli 50

Classic Chicken Salad in a Pita 52

Protein-Packed Peanut Butter and Berry Overnight Oats 53

Second Quick and Easy Three-Day Meal Prep Plan 54

Taco-Stuffed Sweet Potatoes 56

Spicy Tomato-Basil Zoodles with Beef 58

Seasoned Ground Beef 60

Portable Breakfast Protein Boxes 61

« Protein-Packed Peanut Butter and Berry Overnight Oats (page 53)

First Quick and Easy Three-Day Meal Prep Plan

This meal prep was created to show you how you can take one recipe for the main protein and turn it into two different meals. The more meals you can eat out of cooking just once, the more efficient your meal prep will be.

SHOPPING LIST

PANTRY
- Black pepper, freshly ground
- Chia seeds
- Farro
- Honey
- Mayonnaise (made with avocado oil or olive oil)
- Mustard, Dijon
- Oats, old-fashioned
- Oil, avocado
- Peanut butter
- Peanut butter powder, defatted
- Sea salt

CANNED, BOTTLED, PACKAGED, AND PREPARED
- Broth, low-sodium vegetable (3 cups)
- Italian dressing or marinade, fat-free (1 [12-ounce] bottle)
- Pickles, dill, diced (⅓ cup)
- Pita bread, whole-wheat (3)

FRUITS, VEGETABLES, FRESH HERBS, AND SPICES
- Blueberries (1½ cups)
- Broccoli florets (1½ pounds)
- Celery stalks (3)
- Garlic (1 head)
- Lemons (2)
- Onion, red (1)
- Onion, yellow (1)
- Parsley (1 bunch)
- Spinach (3 cups)

PROTEIN
- Chicken breast, boneless, skinless (2 pounds)

DAIRY
- Milk, low-fat 2% (1½ cups)

EQUIPMENT LIST
- Airtight storage containers
- Aluminum foil
- Baking sheets
- Chef's knife
- Cutting board
- Food scale
- Food thermometer
- Grill
- Measuring cups and spoons
- Medium pot
- Mixing bowls
- Parchment paper
- Pint-size Mason jars
- Plastic resealable quart-size bags or plastic wrap

	Breakfast	Lunch	Dinner
DAY 1	Protein-Packed Peanut Butter and Berry Overnight Oats (page 53)	Classic Chicken Salad in a Pita (page 52)	Garlic and Herb Farro with Lemon-Pepper Broccoli (page 50)
DAY 2	Protein-Packed Peanut Butter and Berry Overnight Oats (page 53)	Classic Chicken Salad in a Pita (page 52)	Garlic and Herb Farro with Lemon-Pepper Broccoli (page 50)
DAY 3	Protein-Packed Peanut Butter and Berry Overnight Oats (page 53)	Classic Chicken Salad in a Pita (page 52)	Garlic and Herb Farro with Lemon-Pepper Broccoli (page 50)

STEP-BY-STEP GUIDE

1. Follow the instructions for **Italian Marinated Grilled Chicken** (page 48) to marinate the chicken prior to starting your meal prep.

2. Follow steps 1 through 5 for **Garlic and Herb Farro with Lemon-Pepper Broccoli** (page 50).

3. While the farro and broccoli cook, grill the marinated chicken.

4. Once the farro, broccoli, and grilled chicken are done, portion out 1 cup of cooked farro, 1 portion of broccoli, and 4 ounces of grilled chicken into each of 3 meal prep containers. Refrigerate or freeze the containers, as needed.

5. Complete steps 1 and 2 for **Classic Chicken Salad in a Pita** (page 52).

6. Make **Protein-Packed Peanut Butter and Berry Overnight Oats** (page 53) in its entirety.

Italian Marinated Grilled Chicken

PREP TIME: 1 hour | COOK TIME: 45 minutes

Marinate this chicken to perfection in your favorite flavorful Italian dressing. This recipe forms two meals in one. Pack three portions of the grilled chicken with Garlic and Herb Farro with Lemon-Pepper Broccoli (page 50) and use the remaining chicken to make Classic Chicken Salad in a Pita (page 52).

2 pounds boneless, skinless chicken breast

1½ cups store-bought fat-free Italian dressing or marinade, divided

DAIRY-FREE • DASH • GLUTEN-FREE • MEDITERRANEAN • SOY-FREE

1. In a 9-by-13-inch casserole dish, combine the chicken and dressing, turning the chicken to coat. Cover the dish and refrigerate for at least 1 hour, or up to 24 hours, flipping the chicken in the marinade once or twice.

2. Preheat a grill to 400°F.

3. Remove the chicken from the marinade and place it on the grill. Cook the chicken, turning occasionally, until its internal temperature reaches 165°F.

4. Place 4 ounces of grilled chicken into 3 storage containers.

5. Complete the meal, making Garlic and Herb Farro with Lemon-Pepper Broccoli (page 50). Reserve the remaining chicken for Classic Chicken Salad in a Pita (page 52).

STORAGE TIP: You can freeze the chicken, farro, and broccoli dinner portions. Thaw in the refrigerator overnight and reheat to 165°F.

INGREDIENT TIP: Although this recipe is indicated as gluten-free, if this is a concern for you, check the ingredient packaging to ensure all foods were processed in a completely gluten-free facility.

Per Serving (4 ounces grilled chicken): Calories: 205; Fat: 2g; Carbohydrates: 8g; Fiber: 0g; Protein: 34g; Sodium: 500mg*

*Sodium varies depending on brand of the Italian dressing you use; choose a low-sodium brand if possible.

Garlic *and* Herb Farro *with* Lemon-Pepper Broccoli

PREP TIME: 15 minutes | COOK TIME: 40 minutes

Farro is higher in protein than other grains, but much easier to cook. It's chewy and slightly nutty with a hint of sweetness. The fragrant farro pairs perfectly with the tender yet crisp lemon-pepper broccoli. Broccoli is packed with inflammation-fighting and tumor-suppressing antioxidants and phytochemicals.

2 tablespoons avocado oil, divided

½ sweet yellow onion, chopped

3 garlic cloves, minced

3 cups low-sodium vegetable broth

1 cup farro

½ cup chopped fresh parsley

1½ pounds broccoli florets

2 lemons, 1 halved, 1 cut into wedges

½ teaspoon freshly ground black pepper

¼ teaspoon sea salt

DAIRY-FREE • DASH • GLUTEN-FREE • MEDITERRANEAN • SOY-FREE

1. Preheat the oven to 400°F and line a baking sheet with aluminum foil.

2. In a 6-quart pot over medium heat, heat 1 tablespoon of avocado oil. Add the onion and garlic and cook for 3 to 5 minutes, or until the onion is translucent and tender.

3. Add the broth, farro, and parsley and bring the mixture to a boil. Reduce the heat to maintain a simmer and cook for 20 to 30 minutes until the farro is tender. Drain any excess liquid.

4. While the farro begins cooking, spread the broccoli in a single layer on the prepared sheet and toss it with the remaining 1 tablespoon of avocado oil. Squeeze the 2 lemon halves over the broccoli and season it with pepper and salt.

5. Bake the broccoli for 20 minutes, or until fork-tender.

6. Divide the farro and broccoli among the 3 storage containers containing the grilled chicken (see page 48) and set aside to cool. Add 1 lemon wedge to each container.

> **NEED MORE CALORIES?** Double the recipe or add feta cheese or sliced almonds to toss with the farro salad.

INGREDIENT TIP: Can't find farro? Substitute brown rice following the same directions but decrease the vegetable broth to 2 cups and increase the cooking time to 40 to 50 minutes. Substitute 1 tablespoon dried parsley for fresh parsley.

Although this recipe is indicated as gluten-free, if this is a concern for you, check the ingredient packaging to ensure all foods, especially oats, were processed in a completely gluten-free facility.

Per Serving (⅓ recipe): Calories: 353; Fat: 11g; Carbohydrates: 53g; Fiber: 6g; Protein: 11g; Sodium: 341mg

Classic Chicken Salad in a Pita

PREP TIME: 15 minutes

The leftover Italian Marinated Grilled Chicken (see page 48) takes on a host of new flavors when it's mixed with creamy mayonnaise and crunchy fresh veggies, onion, and herbs to make an irresistible chicken salad for lunch. Stuff it into a pita for a simple portable lunch that tastes great and leaves you feeling satisfied.

2 cups chopped Italian Marinated Grilled Chicken (page 48)

3 celery stalks, chopped

⅓ cup diced dill pickle

¼ cup finely chopped red onion

¼ cup mayonnaise

2 tablespoons Dijon mustard

1 tablespoon fresh parsley

3 cups fresh spinach

3 whole-wheat pitas, halved

DAIRY-FREE • DASH • MEDITERRANEAN • SOY-FREE

1.   In a medium bowl, combine the chicken, celery, pickle, red onion, mayonnaise, mustard, and parsley and stir to mix well. Equally divide the chicken salad among 6 storage containers.

2.   Place ½ cup of spinach on top of each portion of chicken.

3.   Place the pita breads in individual storage bags or containers.

4.   When ready to eat, fill the pita pockets with the spinach and chicken salad.

NEED MORE CALORIES? Double the recipe for the chicken salad and double the portions for each meal. Add avocado slices to the pita pockets before adding the chicken salad.

STORAGE TIP: Classic Chicken Salad in a Pita does not freeze well. Pita bread can be frozen, but chicken salad cannot.

INGREDIENT TIP: The healthiest mayo to use is one made with avocado oil or olive oil.

Per Serving (½ pita stuffed with chicken salad and ½ cup spinach): Calories: 245; Fat: 9g; Carbohydrates: 20g; Fiber: 3g; Protein: 21g; Sodium: 402mg

Protein-Packed Peanut Butter *and* Berry Overnight Oats

PREP TIME: 15 minutes

Creamy, peanut buttery oats with fresh blueberries in every bite is the perfect start to your day. These make-ahead protein-packed overnight oats are a portable breakfast favorite that keeps you full much longer than your typical "instant oats packet."

1½ cups old-fashioned oats

1½ cups low-fat (2%) milk

1½ teaspoons chia seeds

⅓ cup defatted peanut butter powder

3 tablespoons peanut butter

1 tablespoon honey

1½ cups fresh blueberries

DASH • GLUTEN-FREE • MEDITERRANEAN • SOY-FREE • VEGETARIAN

1.   In a large bowl, stir together the oats, milk, chia seeds, peanut butter powder, peanut butter, and honey. Evenly divide the mixture among 3 pint-size Mason jars.

2.   Top each with ½ cup of blueberries. Cover and refrigerate.

3.   Heat for 2 to 3 minutes in the microwave before serving, if you prefer your oats warmed, or enjoy cold.

> **NEED MORE CALORIES?** Double the recipe and eat two portions instead of one. Two portions should still fit in a pint-size Mason jar.

STORAGE TIP: Keep the oats refrigerated for up to 5 days. These can be frozen after the oats have been refrigerated for 24 hours. Reheat to 165°F.

INGREDIENT TIP: Oats are naturally gluten-free, but are sometimes contaminated with gluten during processing. Look for certified gluten-free oats if you need them to gluten-free.

Per Serving (1 oat jar): Calories: 422; Fat: 17g; Carbohydrates: 54g; Fiber: 9g; Protein: 19g; Sodium: 145mg

Second Quick and Easy Three-Day Meal Prep Plan

This week was created to show you that meals don't always have to come from "full recipes." You can piece together a protein, veggie, and carb to make delicious meals with a ton of flavor. Your breakfast will feature a portable bento box meal and lunch and dinner will be made from one protein but with vastly different flavors.

SHOPPING LIST

PANTRY

- Black pepper, freshly ground
- Cinnamon, ground
- Italian seasoning, salt-free
- Oil, avocado
- Peanut butter
- Red pepper flakes
- Sea salt
- Sugar, granulated

CANNED, BOTTLED, PACKAGED, AND PREPARED

- Enchilada sauce or taco sauce (1 cup)
- Tomatoes, crushed, (1 [28-ounce] can)
- Tomato paste (1 tablespoon)

FRUITS, VEGETABLES, FRESH HERBS, AND SPICES

- Apples (3)
- Basil (1 bunch)
- Garlic (1 head)
- Lemon (1)
- Onions, yellow (2)
- Parsley (1 bunch)
- Spinach, baby (4 cups)
- Sweet potatoes (3)
- Zucchini, large (2)

PROTEIN

- Beef, ground 90% lean (2 pounds)
- Eggs, large (6)
- Turkey bacon (6 slices)

DAIRY

- Cheese, goat (4 ounces)

EQUIPMENT LIST

- Airtight storage containers
- Aluminum foil
- Baking sheets
- Chef's knife
- Cutting board
- Dressing containers (2-ounce)
- Food thermometer
- Large skillet
- Measuring cups and spoons
- Mixing bowls
- Saucepan
- Spiralizer

	Breakfast	Lunch	Dinner
DAY 1	Portable Breakfast Protein Boxes (page 61)	Taco-Stuffed Sweet Potatoes (page 56)	Spicy Tomato-Basil Zoodles with Beef (page 58)
DAY 2	Portable Breakfast Protein Boxes (page 61)	Taco-Stuffed Sweet Potatoes (page 56)	Spicy Tomato-Basil Zoodles with Beef (page 58)
DAY 3	Portable Breakfast Protein Boxes (page 61)	Taco-Stuffed Sweet Potatoes (page 56)	Spicy Tomato-Basil Zoodles with Beef (page 58)

STEP-BY-STEP GUIDE

1. Start by getting the sweet potatoes for **Taco-Stuffed Sweet Potatoes** (page 56) in the oven as those take the longest to cook, following the instructions. Set a timer for 20 minutes so you remember to flip them halfway through the cooking time.

2. Start the **Spicy Tomato-Basil Marinara** (see page 58), following steps 1 through 3.

3. On another burner, start the **Seasoned Ground Beef** (page 60), following steps 1 and 2.

4. Prep the zoodles, and divide them into storage containers.

5. Finish cooking the ground beef and finish the marinara. Add the marinara and ground beef to the divided zoodles to finish packing these meals. Finish prepping the sweet potatoes as soon as the sweet potatoes are done baking.

6. Follow the instructions for **Portable Breakfast Protein Boxes** (page 61) in its entirety.

Taco-Stuffed Sweet Potatoes

PREP TIME: 5 minutes | COOK TIME: 1 hour

Sweet potatoes offer more fiber, vitamins, and minerals than white potatoes. Baking sweet potatoes brings out their natural sweetness so each bite is sweet and creamy to the end.

3 sweet potatoes

1 tablespoon avocado oil

½ recipe Seasoned Ground Beef (page 60)

4 cups fresh baby spinach

1 cup enchilada sauce, or taco sauce

DAIRY-FREE • GLUTEN-FREE • SOY-FREE

1.   Preheat the oven to 400°F and line a baking sheet with aluminum foil.

2.   Using a fork, pierce each sweet potato 4 or 5 times and rub them all over with the avocado oil. Place the sweet potatoes on the prepared baking sheet and cook for 45 minutes to 1 hour, or until fork-tender, turning the sweet potatoes over halfway through the baking time. Remove the sweet potatoes from the oven and cut lengthways down the center, stopping before cutting all the way through the potato.

3.   Place 1 sweet potato into each of 3 storage containers and let it cool.

4.   In a large skillet, combine the cooked beef and spinach and stir until the spinach wilts, about 2 minutes.

5. Add the enchilada sauce to the beef, stir, and simmer for
5 minutes.

6. Add one-third of the ground beef–spinach mixture to
each baked sweet potato. Allow it to cool, cover, and refrigerate
the containers.

> **NEED MORE CALORIES?** Drizzle more oil over the sweet
> potatoes or double the amount of ground beef so each
> meal has twice the amount of protein.

STORAGE TIP: Keep refrigerated for up to 3 days, or freeze the
meal in individual glass or freezer-friendly containers. Thaw in
the refrigerator overnight and reheat to 165°F.

INGREDIENT TIP: Although this recipe is indicated as gluten-free,
if this is a concern for you, check the ingredient packaging to
ensure all foods, especially oats, were processed in a completely
gluten-free facility.

Per Serving (1 beef and spinach–stuffed sweet potato): Calories: 428;
Fat: 20g; Carbohydrates: 40g; Fiber: 6g; Protein: 26g; Sodium: 1,082mg

Spicy Tomato-Basil Zoodles *with* Beef

PREP TIME: 15 minutes | COOK TIME: 30 minutes

There is nothing that compares to the fresh flavor of homemade marinara sauce. In this sauce, you'll taste fresh herbs, a little bit of heat from the red pepper flakes, and a slight tang from the goat cheese.

2 tablespoons avocado oil

1 small yellow
onion, chopped

2 garlic cloves, minced

1 tablespoon tomato paste

1 teaspoon red
pepper flakes

1 (28-ounce) can crushed
tomatoes

¼ cup chopped
fresh parsley

¼ cup chopped fresh basil

1 tablespoon salt-free
Italian seasoning

1 teaspoon sugar

½ teaspoon sea salt

¼ teaspoon freshly ground
black pepper

2 large zucchini

4 ounces goat cheese

½ recipe Seasoned Ground
Beef (page 60)

GLUTEN-FREE • SOY-FREE

1.   In a saucepan or deep skillet, heat the avocado oil over medium-high heat. Add the onion and garlic and sauté for 3 to 5 minutes until the onion is translucent and tender.

2.   Stir in the tomato paste and red peppers flakes. Sauté for 1 minute.

3.   Stir in the crushed tomatoes, parsley, basil, Italian seasoning, sugar, salt, and pepper. Simmer the mixture for 20 to 30 minutes—the longer it cooks, the better it will taste.

4.   While the sauce cooks, spiralize the zucchini. If you don't have a spiralizer, chop it into ½-inch half-moon pieces instead of creating zoodles. Equally divide the zucchini among 3 storage containers.

5. Stir the goat cheese into the sauce, stirring until it melts.

6. Pour a ½ cup of sauce over the zucchini in each container and evenly divide the cooked ground beef, placing it on top. Allow it to cool, cover, and refrigerate the containers.

STORAGE TIP: Keep refrigerated for up to 3 days.

INGREDIENT TIP: You will have half of the spicy tomato marinara left over. Freeze the remainder so it's ready the next time you want to make this meal or need marinara sauce!

Not a fan of goat cheese or don't like spicy foods? Omit the goat cheese and red pepper flakes, as desired.

Although this recipe is indicated as gluten-free, if this is a concern for you, check the ingredient packaging to ensure all foods, especially oats, were processed in a completely gluten-free facility.

Per Serving (⅓ recipe): Calories: 452; Fat: 26g; Carbohydrates: 28g; Fiber: 8g; Protein: 30g; Sodium: 1,053mg

Seasoned Ground Beef

PREP TIME: 10 minutes | **COOK TIME:** 20 minutes

This ground beef is anything but plain. You will use lean ground beef to keep the calories in check while ramping up the flavor with garlic, onion, sea salt, and pepper.

1 tablespoon avocado oil

1 small yellow onion, chopped

2 garlic cloves, minced

2 pounds 90% lean ground beef

¼ teaspoon sea salt

¼ teaspoon freshly ground black pepper

DAIRY-FREE • DASH • GLUTEN-FREE • SOY-FREE

1. In a large skillet, heat the avocado oil over medium-high heat. Add the onion and garlic and sauté for 3 to 5 minutes until the onion is translucent and tender.

2. Add the ground beef, season with salt and pepper, and cook until it browns and no pink remains, about 10 minutes.

STORAGE TIP: Freeze the cooked ground beef, once cooled, in a large freezer bag or freezer container. Thaw in the refrigerator overnight and reheat to 165°F.

INGREDIENT TIP: Although this recipe is indicated as gluten-free, if this is a concern for you, check the ingredient packaging to ensure all foods were processed in a completely gluten-free facility.

Per Serving (4 ounces): Calories: 228; Fat: 14g; Carbohydrates: 2g; Fiber: 1g; Protein: 23g; Sodium: 197mg

Portable Breakfast Protein Boxes

PREP TIME: 10 minutes | COOK TIME: 15 minutes

Enjoy this balanced breakfast that gives you a little dose of savory, sweet, salty, and creamy to start your day. Because this does not freeze well, keep the boxes refrigerated and consume within 3 to 5 days of preparing.

6 large eggs

6 turkey bacon slices

3 apples, cored and sliced

1 tablespoon freshly squeezed lemon juice

1 teaspoon ground cinnamon

⅓ cup peanut butter

Pinch sea salt

DAIRY-FREE • DASH • GLUTEN-FREE • MEDITERRANEAN • SOY-FREE

1. In a medium pot, combine the eggs with enough cold water to cover by 1 inch. Place the pot over high heat, cover it, and bring the water to a boil.

2. Once boiling, remove the lid and boil the eggs for 9 minutes.

3. Using a slotted spoon, transfer the eggs to a bowl filled with cold water to cool. Once cool enough to handle, peel the eggs and place 2 eggs in each of the 3 storage containers.

4. In a skillet over medium heat, cook the turkey bacon for 6 minutes. Flip the bacon and cook for 6 minutes more until crispy. Add 2 pieces of cooked bacon to each storage container.

5. In a small bowl, toss the apples, lemon juice, and cinnamon to coat. Add one-third of the apples to each storage container.

6. Place 2 tablespoons of peanut butter into each of 3 (2-ounce) containers and cover. Add them to the meal box, close the lids, and refrigerate.

NEED MORE CALORIES? Add another egg and piece of turkey bacon to increase the protein content. Add another serving of fruit, such as 1 cup of berries, for more carbs.

Per Serving (1 filled box): Calories: 398; Fat: 23g; Carbohydrates: 32g; Fiber: 6g; Protein: 25g; Sodium: 78mg

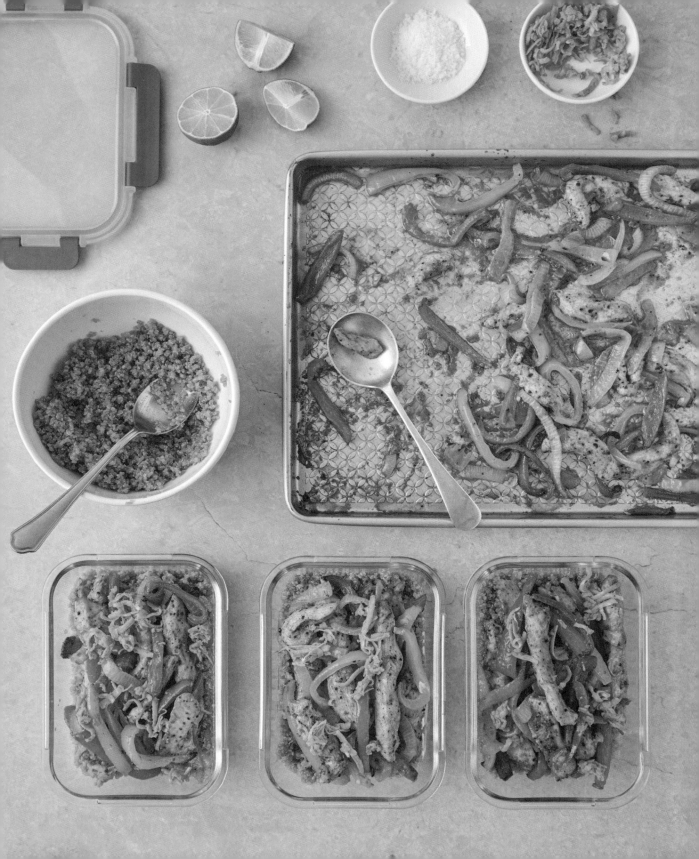

CHAPTER FIVE

Flavor Variety Five-Recipe Meal Preps

First Flavor Variety Five-Day Meal Prep 64

Slow-Cooked Pork Tenderloin with Apples and Carrots 67

Meal Prep Breakfast Sandwiches 69

Easy Sheet Pan Chicken Fajitas 71

Pan-Seared Trout with Tzatziki Sauce, Arugula,
and Quinoa Salad 73

Crunchy Rainbow Salad with Thai Peanut Dressing 75

Second Flavor Variety Five-Day Meal Prep Plan 76

Slow Cooker Three-Bean Chili 79

Mediterranean Lentil Salad with Tahini Dressing 80

High-Protein Egg Salad Boxes 81

Caprese Chicken Pasta with Roasted Tomatoes 82

Turkey, Spinach, and Sweet Potato Breakfast Hash 84

« Easy Sheet Pan Chicken Fajitas (page 71)

First Flavor Variety Five-Day Meal Prep

This week you will prep five recipes but don't be intimidated—you've got this! It will be easier than you think. The recipes vary significantly in flavor, so you'll never get bored with your meals. You'll see we use quinoa in multiple recipes, so you'll only cook it once and then turn it into several meals with varying flavors.

SHOPPING LIST

PANTRY

- Black pepper, freshly ground
- Cayenne pepper
- Cumin, ground
- Garlic powder
- Ginger, ground
- Honey
- Nonstick cooking spray
- Oil, avocado
- Onion powder
- Paprika, smoked
- Peanut butter, creamy
- Quinoa
- Sea salt
- Soy sauce, low-sodium
- Sriracha
- Sugar, granulated
- Vinegar, apple cider
- Vinegar, rice

CANNED, BOTTLED, PACKAGED, AND PREPARED

- Broth, low-sodium vegetable (3½ cups)
- English muffins, 100% whole-grain (6)

FRUITS, VEGETABLES, FRESH HERBS, AND SPICES

- Apple, Gala (1)
- Arugula (4 cups)
- Bell peppers, any color (3)
- Broccoli crowns (2 cups)
- Carrots, baby (1 [1-pound] bag)
- Carrots (5)
- Garlic (1 head)
- Kale, Tuscan (4½ cups)
- Limes (2)
- Onion, white (1)

PROTEIN

- Canadian bacon, precooked (6 slices)
- Chicken breast, boneless, skinless (18 ounces)
- Eggs, large (12)
- Pork tenderloin (1 pound)
- Steelhead trout (2 [8-ounce] fillets)

DAIRY

- Milk, low-fat 2% (¼ cup)
- Cheese, Cheddar, sliced (6 [1-ounce] slices)
- Cheese, Mexican blend, shredded (2 ounces [⅓ cup])
- Tzatziki dressing/sauce (½ cup)

	Breakfast	Lunch	Dinner
DAY 1	Meal Prep Breakfast Sandwiches (page 69)	Pan-Seared Trout with Tzatziki Sauce, Arugula, and Quinoa Salad (page 73)	Slow-Cooked Pork Tenderloin with Apples and Carrots (page 67)
DAY 2	Meal Prep Breakfast Sandwiches (page 69)	Pan-Seared Trout with Tzatziki Sauce, Arugula, and Quinoa Salad (page 73)	Slow-Cooked Pork Tenderloin with Apples and Carrots (page 67)
DAY 3	Meal Prep Breakfast Sandwiches (page 69)	Crunchy Rainbow Salad with Thai Peanut Dressing (page 75)	Easy Sheet Pan Chicken Fajitas (page 71)
DAY 4	Meal Prep Breakfast Sandwiches (page 69)	Crunchy Rainbow Salad with Thai Peanut Dressing (page 75)	Easy Sheet Pan Chicken Fajitas (page 71)
DAY 5	Meal Prep Breakfast Sandwiches (page 69)	Crunchy Rainbow Salad with Thai Peanut Dressing (page 75)	Easy Sheet Pan Chicken Fajitas (page 71)

FROZEN
- Edamame, shelled (3 cups)

EQUIPMENT LIST
- 9-by-13-inch casserole dish
- Airtight storage containers
- Aluminum foil
- Baking sheets
- Chef's knife
- Cutting board
- Food thermometer
- Large skillet
- Measuring cups and spoons
- Medium pot
- Mixing bowls
- Parchment paper
- Resealable quart-size plastic bags or plastic wrap
- Silicone egg muffin holders
- Slow cooker

continued

STEP-BY-STEP GUIDE

1. Complete steps 1 through 5 of **Slow-Cooked Pork Tenderloin with Apples and Carrots** (page 67).

2. Preheat the oven to 375°F.

3. Next, complete steps 1 through 4 of **Meal Prep Breakfast Sandwiches** (page 69).

4. While the eggs bake, start the **Easy Sheet Pan Chicken Fajitas** (page 71) so when the eggs come out of the oven, the fajitas can go in.

5. Complete steps 1 through 6 of the fajita recipe (omitting the quinoa step).

6. There is quinoa in both the quinoa salad served with trout and the fajitas recipe. In a medium pot over high, bring 4 cups vegetable broth to a boil. Add 1½ cups quinoa, rinsed well, reduce the heat to maintain a simmer, cover the pot, and cook for 15 minutes, or until all the liquid is absorbed. The finished quinoa will look fluffy.

7. When the eggs come out of the oven, remove them (using the parchment paper) from the casserole dish. Cut them into squares and refrigerate to cool completely.

8. While the fajitas are in the oven, the quinoa cooks, and the eggs cool, complete steps 1 through 4 for **Pan-Seared Trout with Tzatziki Sauce, Arugula, and Quinoa Salad** (page 73). Once the fish is done, refrigerate it to cool.

9. When the trout is done, finish the egg muffins.

10. Finish the fajitas recipe, portioning everything.

11. When the trout is cooled, finish the arugula and quinoa salad.

12. Make the **Crunchy Rainbow Salad with Thai Peanut Dressing** (page 75).

13. Portion the pork tenderloin recipe when it's done cooking.

Slow-Cooked Pork Tenderloin *with* Apples *and* Carrots

PREP TIME: 15 minutes | COOK TIME: 4 to 6 hours

This is a juicy pork tenderloin, panfried to lock in flavor then slow cooked to tender perfection with sweet apple and carrots.

1 pound pork tenderloin

¼ teaspoon sea salt

¼ teaspoon freshly ground black pepper

1 tablespoon avocado oil

1 Gala apple, cored and halved

3 garlic cloves, halved

1 cup low-sodium vegetable broth

¼ cup low-sodium soy sauce

1 teaspoon apple cider vinegar

1 (1-pound) bag baby carrots

DAIRY-FREE • DASH

1. Season the pork tenderloin all over with salt and pepper.

2. In a skillet, heat the avocado oil for 1 minute over medium-high heat. Add the pork and sear it for 2 to 3 minutes. Flip the tenderloin and sear the other side for 2 to 3 minutes more.

3. Remove the pork from the skillet and cut 12 to 15 small slits on each side of the tenderloin. Cut half the apple into very thin slices. Place the garlic cloves and apple slices into the slits in the pork tenderloin.

4. In a slow cooker, combine the vegetable broth, soy sauce, and vinegar.

continued

5.   Place the pork in the slow cooker. Chop the remaining half apple and spread it evenly around the pork. Add the carrots to the slow cooker.

6.   Cover the cooker and cook on high heat for 4 to 6 hours until the pork reaches an internal temperature of 145°F and the vegetables are soft.

NEED MORE CALORIES? Double the pork portion and increase the slow cooker time by 1 hour for every additional pound of pork. You don't need to increase the liquids unless you go above 3 pounds of meat total.

STORAGE TIP: Freeze the pork and vegetables in individual portions. Thaw in the refrigerator overnight and reheat to 165°F.

INGREDIENT TIP: To make this recipe gluten-free and soy-free, use coconut aminos instead of the soy sauce.

Per Serving (½ recipe): Calories: 495; Fat: 13g; Carbohydrates: 42g; Fiber: 10g; Protein: 46g; Sodium: 500mg

Meal Prep Breakfast Sandwiches

PREP TIME: 10 minutes | COOK TIME: 25 minutes

A piping hot, cheesy breakfast sandwich is the perfect way to start your day. These breakfast sandwiches are a fast and delicious option to get those filling proteins and nutrients for breakfast.

Nonstick cooking spray

12 large eggs

¼ cup low-fat (2%) milk

½ teaspoon sea salt

¼ teaspoon freshly ground black pepper

2 cups chopped broccoli

6 whole-grain English muffins, split

6 precooked Canadian bacon slices

6 Cheddar cheese slices

SOY-FREE

1. Preheat the oven to 375°F. Line a 9-by-13-inch casserole dish with parchment paper and coat it with cooking spray.

2. In a small bowl, whisk the eggs, milk, salt, and pepper. Pour the eggs into the prepared dish. Add the broccoli to the dish, spreading it evenly.

3. Bake the casserole for 20 to 25 minutes until the top browns and the eggs are just set.

4. Remove the dish from the oven, lift the parchment paper out of the dish to remove the casserole, and cut it into six squares. Let cool completely.

5. On the bottom half of each English muffin, layer 1 egg square, 1 slice of Canadian bacon, and 1 slice of cheese. Add the top of the English muffin to each. Wrap the sandwiches in parchment paper or aluminum foil to close.

continued

6. To reheat in the oven: Preheat the oven to 425°F. Place the wrapped sandwich in the oven for 25 to 35 minutes, or, if frozen, for 1 hour.

7. To reheat in the microwave: Remove the foil or parchment wrapping and wrap the sandwich in a paper towel and fresh parchment paper. Place it in the microwave and heat for 2 to 3 minutes on 60 percent power, flipping every minute, or, if frozen, for 5 to 7 minutes, flipping every 2 minutes.

NEED MORE CALORIES? Eat two sandwiches or add one extra slice of Canadian bacon and ½ of an avocado (added the day you eat it).

Per Serving (1 sandwich): Calories: 446; Fat: 22g; Carbohydrates: 31g; Fiber: 4g; Protein: 14g; Sodium: 1,052mg

Easy Sheet Pan Chicken Fajitas

PREP TIME: 15 minutes | **COOK TIME:** 25 minutes

These sheet pan fajitas are a mouthwatering combination of juicy chicken, fresh bell pepper, and savory onion. This sizzling combo is served over a bed of fluffy quinoa and topped with melting cheese.

1½ cups low-sodium vegetable broth

½ cup quinoa, rinsed well

1 teaspoon onion powder

1 teaspoon garlic powder

¼ teaspoon cayenne pepper

1 teaspoon smoked paprika

½ teaspoon sugar

1 teaspoon ground cumin

½ teaspoon sea salt

18 ounces boneless, skinless chicken breast, cut into ½-inch strips

3 bell peppers, any color, cut into ½-inch strips

1 white onion, sliced

1 tablespoon avocado oil

⅓ cup shredded Mexican cheese

Juice of 2 limes

GLUTEN-FREE • MEDITERRANEAN • SOY-FREE

1.   Preheat the oven to 400°F and line a baking sheet with aluminum foil.

2.   In a medium pot over high heat, bring the broth to a boil.

3.   Add the quinoa, reduce the heat to maintain a simmer, cover the pot, and cook for 15 minutes, or until all the liquid is absorbed. The finished quinoa will look fluffy.

4.   While the quinoa cooks, in a large resealable bag, combine the onion powder, garlic powder, cayenne, paprika, sugar, cumin, and salt.

5.   Add the chicken, bell peppers, onion, and avocado oil. Close the bag and shake to coat the chicken well. Pour the chicken and vegetables onto the prepared baking sheet and spread them out evenly.

6.   Bake for 20 to 25 minutes, or until the chicken's internal temperature reaches 165°F and the vegetables are soft.

continued

7.   Adjust the oven to broil and cook for 5 minutes more.

8.   Into each of 3 storage containers, place about 1 cup of quinoa. Divide the chicken and vegetable mixture atop the quinoa. Add about 2 tablespoons of Mexican cheese and 1 tablespoon of freshly squeezed lime juice to each container. Cover and refrigerate.

> **NEED MORE CALORIES?** Double the fajitas portion (chicken, veggies, and seasonings) and add 2 tablespoons more cheese.

STORAGE TIP: Freeze the meal in individual portions. Thaw in the refrigerator overnight and reheat to 165°F.

INGREDIENT TIP: Some quinoa comes prerinsed, and other products do not. If it's not prerinsed, place the quinoa in a fine-mesh strainer and rinse it until the water runs clear.

Although this recipe is indicated as gluten-free, if this is a concern for you, check the ingredient packaging to ensure all foods, especially oats, were processed in a completely gluten-free facility.

Per Serving (⅓ recipe): Calories: 455; Fat: 15g; Carbohydrates: 40g; Fiber: 5g; Protein: 45g; Sodium: 589mg

Pan-Seared Trout *with* Tzatziki Sauce, Arugula, *and* Quinoa Salad

PREP TIME: 10 minutes | **COOK TIME:** 20 minutes

Arugula has a naturally peppery taste that perfectly complements this crispy panfried trout slathered with creamy and slightly tangy tzatziki sauce.

1 cup low-sodium vegetable broth

½ cup quinoa, rinsed well

2 (8-ounce) steelhead trout fillets

½ teaspoon sea salt

½ teaspoon freshly ground black pepper

1 tablespoon avocado oil

4 cups arugula

½ cup store-bought tzatziki sauce

GLUTEN-FREE • MEDITERRANEAN • SOY-FREE

1. In a medium pot over high heat, bring the broth to a boil. Add the quinoa, reduce the heat to maintain a simmer, cover the pot, and cook for 15 minutes, or until all the liquid is absorbed. The finished quinoa will look fluffy.

2. While the quinoa cooks, season the trout on both sides with salt and pepper.

3. In a nonstick skillet over medium heat, heat the avocado oil. Add the fish and cook for 3 to 4 minutes. Flip and cook the other side for 4 to 5 minutes more, or until the fish is cooked through and flakes easily with a fork. Remove the fish from the skillet and let it cool for 10 minutes.

4. Into each of 2 storage containers, place 1 cooled fish fillet and 2 cups of arugula.

5. Into each of two small storage containers, place ¼ cup tzatziki and seal the lids.

6. Once the quinoa is done, let it cool. Add half the cooled quinoa (about ⅔ cup) to each meal prep container.

continued

7. To reheat, remove the fish from the container, wrap it in a paper towel, and heat for 30 seconds to 1 minute or until hot. (See pages 23–24 for tips on reheating fish.)

8. Add the hot fish to the salad and drizzle with tzatziki.

NEED MORE CALORIES? Double the trout portions and seasoning.

INGREDIENT TIP: Some quinoa comes prerinsed, and other products do not. If it's not prerinsed, place the quinoa in a fine-mesh strainer and rinse it until the water runs clear.

Although this recipe is indicated as gluten-free, if this is a concern for you, check the ingredient packaging to ensure all foods, especially oats, were processed in a completely gluten-free facility.

Per Serving (½ recipe): Calories: 555; Fat: 27g; Carbohydrates: 34g; Fiber: 4g; Protein: 43g; Sodium: 783mg

Crunchy Rainbow Salad
with Thai Peanut Dressing

PREP TIME: 15 minutes

This crunchy salad is drizzled with a creamy Thai peanut dressing with a bit of spice. Carrots, kale, and edamame create a colorful antioxidant-rich combination bursting with flavor.

4½ cups chopped Lacinato kale

1½ cups shredded carrot

3 cups frozen shelled edamame

6 to 8 tablespoons water, divided

⅓ cup creamy peanut butter

2 tablespoons rice vinegar

2 tablespoons low-sodium soy sauce

½ teaspoon honey

1 tablespoon Sriracha

½ teaspoon ground ginger

¼ teaspoon garlic powder

DAIRY-FREE • MEDITERRANEAN • VEGETARIAN

1.　In a bowl, toss together the kale and carrot. Divide the mixture among 3 storage containers.

2.　In a small microwave-safe bowl, combine the edamame and 2 tablespoons of water. Cover the bowl and microwave it on high power for 1 to 2 minutes to thaw the edamame. Drain. Add 1 cup of edamame to each storage container.

3.　In a small bowl, whisk the peanut butter, vinegar, soy sauce, honey, Sriracha, ginger, garlic powder, and enough of the remaining 4 to 6 tablespoons of water to get your desired consistency. Divide the dressing among 3 small (2-ounce) dressing containers, close the lids, and store with the salad.

NEED MORE CALORIES? Double the portions of edamame and add some peanuts on top before serving.

STORAGE TIP: Keep the salad refrigerated for 3 to 5 days. Do not freeze. Add the dressing just before eating.

INGREDIENT TIP: To make this recipe gluten-free and soy-free, use coconut aminos instead of the soy sauce.

Per Serving (⅓ recipe): Calories: 431; Fat: 24g; Carbohydrates: 33g; Fiber: 14g; Protein: 30g; Sodium: 740mg

Second Flavor Variety Five-Day Meal Prep Plan

Now that you've got one five-recipe meal prep under your belt you are probably feeling a lot more confident. Keep that confidence going into this week. You'll use a similar process this week to make your meal prep as efficient and quick as possible.

SHOPPING LIST

PANTRY

- Bay leaves
- Black pepper, freshly ground
- Chili powder
- Cinnamon, ground
- Italian seasoning, salt-free
- Lentils, brown (¾ cup dried)
- Maple syrup, pure
- Mustard, Dijon
- Oil, avocado
- Oil, coconut
- Pickles, dill
- Sea salt
- Tahini
- Vinegar, apple cider

CANNED, BOTTLED, PACKAGED, AND PREPARED

- Balsamic glaze (3 tablespoons)
- Beans, black, no-salt-added (1 [15-ounce] can)
- Beans, great northern, no-salt-added (1 [15-ounce] can)
- Beans, red kidney, no-salt-added (1 [15-ounce] can)
- Broth, low-sodium chicken (1 cup)
- Marinara sauce (2 cups)
- Gluten-free whole grain crackers (1 [4.25-ounce] box)
- Pasta, whole-grain bow-tie (1½ cups, or 3 ounces dried)
- Tomato sauce (1 [15-ounce] can)

FRUITS, VEGETABLES, FRESH HERBS, AND SPICES

- Basil (1 bunch)
- Bell pepper, green (1)
- Bell peppers, orange (3)
- Cucumber, English (1)
- Garlic (1 head)
- Jalapeño pepper (1)
- Kale, Lacinato (6 cups)
- Lemon (1)
- Onion, red, small (1)
- Onion, sweet (1)
- Onion, yellow (1)
- Parsley (1 bunch)
- Spinach, baby (6 cups)
- Sweet potatoes (2)
- Tomatoes, cherry (5 cups)

PROTEIN

- Chicken breast, boneless, skinless (1 pound)
- Eggs, large (6)
- Turkey breakfast sausage, ground (1¾ pounds)
- Turkey or chicken, ground (1½ pounds)

	Breakfast	Lunch	Dinner
DAY 1	Turkey, Spinach, and Sweet Potato Breakfast Hash (page 84)	High-Protein Egg Salad Boxes (page 81)	Caprese Chicken Pasta with Roasted Tomatoes (page 82)
DAY 2	Turkey, Spinach, and Sweet Potato Breakfast Hash (page 84)	High-Protein Egg Salad Boxes (page 81)	Caprese Chicken Pasta with Roasted Tomatoes (page 82)
DAY 3	Turkey, Spinach, and Sweet Potato Breakfast Hash (page 84)	Mediterranean Lentil Salad with Tahini Dressing (page 80)	Slow Cooker Three-Bean Chili (page 79)
DAY 4	Turkey, Spinach, and Sweet Potato Breakfast Hash (page 84)	Mediterranean Lentil Salad with Tahini Dressing (page 80)	Slow Cooker Three-Bean Chili (page 79)
DAY 5	Turkey, Spinach, and Sweet Potato Breakfast Hash (page 84)	Mediterranean Lentil Salad with Tahini Dressing (page 80)	Slow Cooker Three-Bean Chili (page 79)

DAIRY

- Cheese, fat-free cottage (8 ounces)
- Cheese, feta, crumbled (2 ounces [⅓ cup])
- Cheese, Mexican blend, shredded (3 ounces [¾ cup])
- Cheese, whole-milk mozzarella (2 ounces)

EQUIPMENT LIST

- Airtight storage containers
- Aluminum foil
- Baking sheets
- Chef's knife
- Cutting board
- Food thermometer
- Large skillet

continued

- Measuring cups and spoons
- Mixing bowls
- Parchment paper
- Pots (3)
- Resealable plastic quart-size bags or plastic wrap
- Saucepan
- Silicone egg muffin holders or baking sheet
- Slow cooker

STEP-BY-STEP GUIDE

1. Prepare the **Slow Cooker Three-Bean Chili** (page 79) and set it to cook.

2. Make the lentils for the **Mediterranean Lentil Salad with Tahini Dressing** (page 80) on a back burner so they are out of the way; they will take 30 minutes to cook fully.

3. Hard-boil the eggs for **High-Protein Egg Salad Boxes** (page 81) while the lentils cook.

4. Start the pasta for **Caprese Chicken Pasta with Roasted Tomatoes** (page 82) and complete steps 1 through 4 of the recipe.

5. When the eggs are done, cool them in an ice water bath and make the egg salad. Keep an eye on the chicken in the oven and the lentils and pasta on the stove.

6. Finish the egg salad boxes.

7. When the pasta is done, finish the caprese chicken recipe.

8. When the lentils are done, finish the lentil salad recipe.

9. Make the **Turkey, Spinach, and Sweet Potato Breakfast Hash** (page 84) in its entirety.

Slow Cooker Three-Bean Chili

PREP TIME: 15 minutes | COOK TIME: 4 to 6 hours

This slow cooker meal is filled with fiber-rich beans, filling protein, and sweet chili flavor. It's very freezer friendly so you can make a big batch and eat it over the weeks to come.

1 tablespoon avocado oil

1 yellow onion, chopped

1½ pounds ground turkey, or chicken

1 (15-ounce) can no-salt-added red kidney beans, drained and rinsed

1 (15-ounce) can no-salt-added black beans, drained and rinsed

1 (15-ounce) can no-salt-added great northern beans, drained and rinsed

1 (15-ounce) can no-salt-added diced Roma tomatoes

1 (15-ounce) can tomato sauce

1 cup low-sodium chicken broth

1 green bell pepper, chopped

1 jalapeño pepper, seeded and chopped

2 to 4 tablespoons chili powder

¾ cup shredded Mexican cheese blend

DASH • GLUTEN-FREE • MEDITERRANEAN • SOY-FREE

1. In a skillet, heat the avocado oil over medium heat. Add the onion and cook for 1 minute until softened. Add the ground turkey and cook for about 10 minutes until fully cooked and no longer pink. Transfer the turkey and onion to a slow cooker.

2. Add the kidney, black, and great northern beans, tomatoes and their juices, tomato sauce, chicken broth, green bell pepper, jalapeño, and chili powder.

3. Cover the cooker and cook on high heat for 4 to 6 hours, or on low heat for 6 to 8 hours. Divide the chili among 6 storage containers and refrigerate.

4. Once the chili is cooled, top each with 2 tablespoons of Mexican cheese, cover the containers, and return them to the refrigerator.

NEED MORE CALORIES? Eat two portions! Add more toppings, such as avocado, sour cream, or more cheese!

STORAGE TIP: Freeze the chili in individual portions. Thaw in the refrigerator overnight and reheat to 165°F.

Per Serving (⅙ recipe): Calories: 463; Fat: 18g; Carbohydrates: 41g; Fiber: 16g; Protein: 37g; Sodium: 389mg

Mediterranean Lentil Salad
with Tahini Dressing

PREP TIME: 15 minutes | COOK TIME: 30 minutes

High in protein and fiber, lentils are delicious in this crunchy lemony salad with a creamy tahini dressing. Because this does not freeze well, keep refrigerated for up to 5 days.

¾ cup dried brown
    lentils, rinsed

2 bay leaves

3 tablespoons tahini

1½ tablespoons pure
    maple syrup

1 tablespoon freshly
    squeezed lemon juice

1 teaspoon apple
    cider vinegar

⅛ teaspoon sea salt

3 cups cherry
    tomatoes, halved

1 English cucumber, cut into
    ½-inch pieces

⅓ cup crumbled feta cheese

3 tablespoons chopped
    red onion

6 cups chopped
    Lacinato kale

1 tablespoon chopped
    fresh basil

1 tablespoon chopped
    fresh parsley

DASH • GLUTEN-FREE • MEDITERRANEAN • SOY-FREE • VEGETARIAN

1. In a large pot over high heat, combine the lentils, bay leaves, and 2¼ cups water. Bring the lentils to a boil, cover the pot, reduce the heat to maintain a simmer, and cook for 20 to 30 minutes until the lentils are tender. Remove and discard the bay leaves. Drain any excess liquid from the lentils and set them aside to cool.

2. In a small bowl, whisk the tahini, maple syrup, lemon juice, vinegar, and salt with ½ cup warm water until combined. You may have to add more warm water until the dressing thins enough to your desired consistency. Divide the dressing among 3 large Mason jars.

3. Into each jar, on top of the dressing, layer 1 cup of lentils, 1 cup of cherry tomatoes, one-third of the cucumber, about 2 tablespoons of feta cheese, and 1 tablespoon of red onion. Top each with 2 cups of kale and 1 teaspoon each of basil and parsley. Cover and refrigerate.

4. When you are ready to eat, shake the container to coat the salad ingredients with the dressing on the bottom.

NEED MORE CALORIES? Double the amount of feta cheese.

Per Serving (1 jar): Calories: 448; Fat: 13g; Carbohydrates: 64g; Fiber: 13g; Protein: 23g; Sodium: 425mg

High-Protein Egg Salad Boxes

PREP TIME: 15 minutes

This creamy egg salad is great with sea salty crackers and fresh crunchy bell peppers. Swapping cottage cheese for mayonnaise significantly increases the protein and decreases the fat in this recipe. If you have three-compartment storage containers, use them here.

6 hard-boiled eggs, peeled and chopped

1 cup fat-free cottage cheese

2 tablespoons Dijon mustard

⅓ cup diced dill pickle

Sea salt

Freshly ground black pepper

30 gluten-free whole grain crackers

3 cups orange bell pepper strips

MEDITERRANEAN • SOY-FREE • VEGETARIAN

1. In a small bowl, combine the eggs, cottage cheese, mustard, and pickle and season with salt and pepper. Gently stir to mix. Divide the egg salad among 3 small storage containers.

2. Divide the crackers among 3 individual storage containers or resealable bags and the bell peppers into 3 more containers. Refrigerate with the egg salad.

NEED MORE CALORIES? Eat two portions!

STORAGE TIP: Do not freeze this. Refrigerate the egg salad and peppers for 3 to 5 days.

Per Serving (1 box): Calories: 292; Fat: 10g; Carbohydrates: 30g; Fiber: 2g; Protein: 18g; Sodium: 720mg

Caprese Chicken Pasta *with* Roasted Tomatoes

PREP TIME: 10 minutes | **COOK TIME:** 30 minutes

Although pasta isn't typically thought of as a weight-loss food, when eaten in balance with protein and vegetables, it absolutely can be. This whole-grain pasta is tossed with sweet marinara sauce, juicy chicken, and tomatoes and baked to finish.

1½ cups whole-wheat bow-tie pasta (3 ounces dried)

1 pound boneless, skinless chicken breast

1 teaspoon salt-free Italian seasoning

¼ teaspoon sea salt

¼ teaspoon freshly ground black pepper

1 tablespoon avocado oil

2 cups halved cherry tomatoes

2 cups marinara sauce

2 ounces whole-milk mozzarella cheese, sliced

3 tablespoons balsamic glaze

3 tablespoons chopped fresh basil

DASH • MEDITERRANEAN • SOY-FREE

1. Preheat the oven to 400°F.

2. Bring a medium pot of water to a boil over high heat and cook the pasta according to the package directions until al dente. Drain the pasta, rinse it, return it to the pot, and set aside.

3. Season the chicken all over with Italian seasoning, salt, and pepper.

4. In an oven-safe skillet, heat the avocado oil over medium-high heat. Add the chicken and cook for 2 to 3 minutes per side. Add the cherry tomatoes to the skillet and transfer it to the oven. Cook for 10 to 15 minutes, or until the chicken reaches an internal temperature of 165°F.

5. Add the marinara sauce to the pasta and stir to coat. Divide the pasta among 3 storage containers.

6. When the chicken is done, turn the oven to broil.

7. Top each chicken breast with some mozzarella cheese and broil for 3 to 5 minutes until it melts.

8. Place 1 chicken breast on top of each bed of pasta. Divide the cooked cherry tomatoes over each. Drizzle each serving with 1 tablespoon of balsamic glaze and sprinkle with fresh basil.

NEED MORE CALORIES? Eat two portions or just double the amount of chicken in your portion.

STORAGE TIP: This recipe can be frozen in individual portions. Thaw in the refrigerator overnight and reheat to minimum of 165°F.

Per Serving (⅓ recipe): Calories: 499; Fat: 16g; Carbohydrates: 45g; Fiber: 3g; Protein: 46g; Sodium: 352mg

Turkey, Spinach, *and* Sweet Potato Breakfast Hash

PREP TIME: 10 minutes | COOK TIME: 25 minutes

This savory breakfast sausage hash amps up the nutrition with crispy sweet potatoes and sautéed spinach. Made with lean turkey sausage and lightly sweetened with maple syrup and cinnamon, this warming hash tastes great reheated from fresh or frozen, making it a meal prep star.

2 tablespoons coconut oil, divided

½ sweet onion, chopped

2 garlic cloves, minced

1¾ pounds ground turkey breakfast sausage

3 cups cubed (½-inch pieces) sweet potato

1 tablespoon pure maple syrup

1 teaspoon ground cinnamon

6 cups fresh baby spinach

DAIRY-FREE • DASH • GLUTEN-FREE • MEDITERRANEAN • SOY-FREE

1. In a large skillet, heat 1 tablespoon of coconut oil over medium heat. Add the onion and garlic. Cover the skillet and sauté for 2 to 3 minutes until the onion is translucent and tender.

2. Add the sausage and sauté for about 10 minutes until fully cooked and no longer pink. Remove the sausage and onion mixture from the skillet and set aside.

3. Return the skillet to medium heat and heat the remaining 1 tablespoon of coconut oil. Add the sweet potato and cook for 5 minutes. Cover the skillet and cook for 5 minutes more, or until the sweet potatoes are fork-tender. If they start to burn, add 1 to 2 tablespoons of water to the skillet, cover the skillet, and let them steam until done.

4. Stir in the maple syrup and cinnamon.

5. Stir in the spinach until just wilted. Return the cooked turkey sausage and onion mixture to the pan and mix well. Divide the hash among 6 storage containers. Eat a serving today and refrigerate the rest for meals during the week.

NEED MORE CALORIES? Eat two portions!

STORAGE TIP: This recipe can be frozen in individual portions. Thaw it in the refrigerator overnight and reheat to 165°F.

INGREDIENT TIP: Although this recipe is indicated as gluten-free, if this is a concern for you, check the ingredient packaging to ensure all foods were processed in a completely gluten-free facility.

Per Serving (⅙ recipe): Calories: 272; Fat: 13g; Carbohydrates: 19g; Fiber: 3g; Protein: 6g; Sodium: 142mg

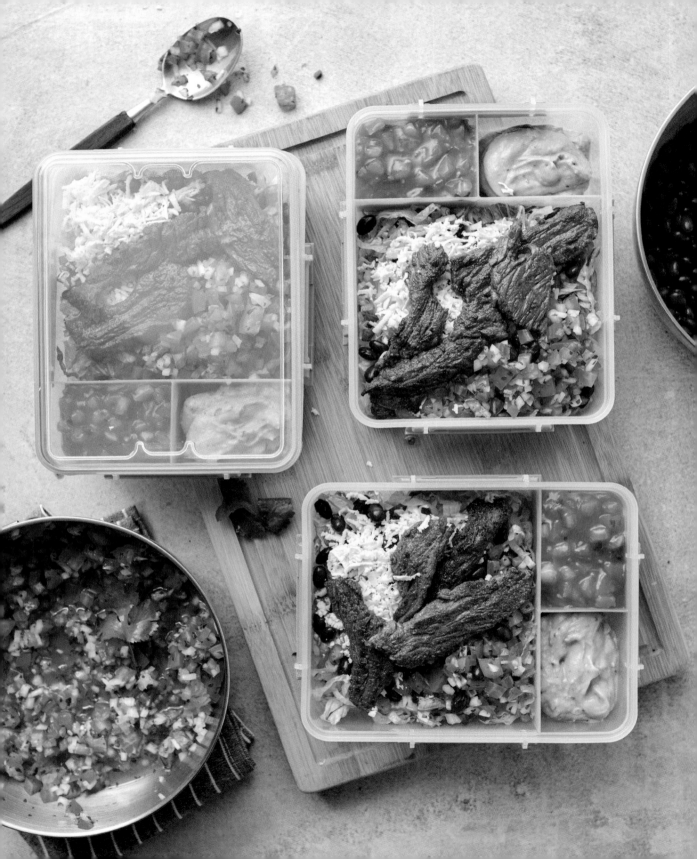

CHAPTER SIX

Superefficient Six-Recipe Meal Preps

First Five-Day Superefficient Prep Plan 88

  Slow Cooker BBQ Chicken 91

  Roasted Sweet Potatoes and Cauliflower 92

  Steak Burrito Bowls 94

  Custom Mini Quiches 96

  Sheet Pan Hummus Chicken and Zucchini 98

  Peanut Butter Chocolate Energy Balls 99

Second Five-Day Superefficient Prep Plan 100

  Slow Cooker Garlic-Parmesan Chicken 103

  Stuffed Bell Peppers 104

  Easy Layered Enchilada Casserole 105

  Chimichurri Shrimp Skewers 107

  Tuna Salad Wraps 108

  Greek Yogurt Blueberry Bites 109

« Steak Burrito Bowls (page 94)

First Five-Day Superefficient Prep Plan

This meal plan is designed to teach you to be superefficient at meal prep. You will prepare six recipes in just a few short hours. And because all your meals will be done for the week, you'll have more time to do what you need and want to do during the week and still eat healthy.

SHOPPING LIST

PANTRY

- Black pepper, freshly ground
- Cayenne pepper
- Chile pepper, ground
- Chili powder
- Flaxseed, ground
- Garlic powder
- Maple syrup, pure
- Nonstick cooking spray
- Oats, rolled
- Oil, avocado
- Onion powder
- Oregano
- Paprika, smoked
- Paprika, sweet
- Peanut butter, natural
- Protein powder, chocolate
- Rice, brown
- Sea salt
- Sugar, granulated
- Vinegar, apple cider

CANNED, BOTTLED, PACKAGED, AND PREPARED

- Barbecue sauce, low-sugar gluten-free (1 [24-ounce] bottle)
- Beans, black, no-salt-added (1 [15-ounce] can)
- Guacamole (⅓ cup)
- Hummus (½ cup)
- Pico de gallo (¾ cup)
- Salsa (1 [8-ounce] jar)

FRUITS, VEGETABLES, FRESH HERBS, AND SPICES

- Bell pepper, red (1)
- Broccoli (1 small crown)
- Cauliflower (2 heads)
- Grapes (6 cups)
- Lettuce, romaine (2 heads)
- Mushrooms (½ cup)
- Parsley (1 bunch)
- Sweet potato (4)
- Zucchini (2)

PROTEIN

- Chicken breast, boneless, skinless (4 pounds)
- Flank steak (1 pound)

DAIRY AND EGGS

- Cheese, Cheddar, shredded (1 ounce [¼ cup])
- Cheese, Mexican blend, shredded (3 ounces [¾ cup])
- Cheese, mozzarella, shredded (1 ounce [¼ cup])
- Cheese, Swiss, shredded (1 ounce [¼ cup])
- Egg whites, liquid (2 cups)
- Eggs, large (6)

	Breakfast	**Lunch**	**Dinner**	**Snack**
DAY 1	Custom Mini Quiches (page 96)	Steak Burrito Bowls (page 94)	Slow Cooker BBQ Chicken with Roasted Sweet Potatoes and Cauliflower (pages 91 and 92)	Peanut Butter Chocolate Energy Balls (page 99)
DAY 2	Custom Mini Quiches (page 96)	Steak Burrito Bowls (page 94)	Slow Cooker BBQ Chicken with Roasted Sweet Potatoes and Cauliflower (pages 91 and 92)	Peanut Butter Chocolate Energy Balls (page 99)
DAY 3	Custom Mini Quiches (page 96)	Steak Burrito Bowls (page 94)	Slow Cooker BBQ Chicken with Roasted Sweet Potatoes and Cauliflower (pages 91 and 92)	Peanut Butter Chocolate Energy Balls (page 99)
DAY 4	Custom Mini Quiches (page 96)	Sheet Pan Hummus Chicken and Zucchini (page 98)	Slow Cooker BBQ Chicken with Roasted Sweet Potatoes and Cauliflower (pages 91 and 92)	Peanut Butter Chocolate Energy Balls (page 99)
DAY 5	Custom Mini Quiches (page 96)	Sheet Pan Hummus Chicken and Zucchini (page 98)	Slow Cooker BBQ Chicken with Roasted Sweet Potatoes and Cauliflower (pages 91 and 92)	Peanut Butter Chocolate Energy Balls (page 99)

continued

EQUIPMENT LIST

- Airtight storage containers
- Aluminum foil
- Baking sheets
- Cast iron skillet
- Chef's knife
- Cutting board
- Food thermometer
- Large skillet
- Measuring cups and spoons
- Mixing bowls
- Parchment paper
- Resealable quart-size plastic bags or plastic wrap
- Silicone egg muffin holders or baking sheet
- Slow cooker

STEP-BY-STEP GUIDE

1. Preheat the oven to 400°F.

2. Prepare the **Slow Cooker BBQ Chicken** (page 91).

3. Complete steps 1 through 4 to begin the **Roasted Sweet Potatoes and Cauliflower** (page 92) and place it in the oven.

4. While the veggies roast, complete the **Steak Burrito Bowls** (page 94).

5. Begin prepping **Custom Mini Quiches** (page 96) so they are ready to go into the oven when the veggies come out. Complete steps 1 through 4 and, when the sweet potatoes and cauliflower are done cooking, reduce the oven temperature to 375°F to cook the quiches.

6. Prepare the **Sheet Pan Hummus Chicken and Zucchini** (page 98) to go into the oven when the mini quiches are done. Complete steps 1 through 3 and, when the quiches are done, increase the oven temperature to 425°F and cook the chicken.

7. Portion out the roasted veggies.

8. Make the **Peanut Butter Chocolate Energy Balls** (page 99).

9. Finish the hummus chicken recipe.

10. When the barbecue chicken is done, complete the remaining steps and portion it.

Slow Cooker BBQ Chicken

PREP TIME: 10 minutes | COOK TIME: 4 to 6 hours

Cooking barbecue chicken in the slow cooker creates moist, delicious chicken out of lean cuts such as the breast. Barbecue can be healthy and weight-loss friendly if you choose a low-sugar barbecue sauce.

3 pounds boneless, skinless chicken breast

1 (24-ounce) bottle low-sugar gluten-free barbecue sauce

2 teaspoons apple cider vinegar

DAIRY-FREE • DASH • GLUTEN-FREE • MEDITERRANEAN • SOY-FREE

1. In a slow cooker, combine the chicken and enough water to cover it. Cover the cooker and cook on high heat for 4 to 6 hours, or on low heat for 6 to 8 hours.

2. Drain the water and transfer the chicken to a bowl. Using two forks, shred the chicken.

3. Return the shredded chicken to the slow cooker and add half the barbecue sauce and mix well to combine.

4. In a small bowl, stir together the remaining barbecue and vinegar and drizzle it over the chicken. Divide the chicken among 8 storage containers. Refrigerate 5 containers for this week's meal plan and freeze the remaining for future meals.

NEED MORE CALORIES? Eat two portions of meat and top your meal with ranch dressing.

STORAGE TIP: Freeze the chicken in one big batch or in individual portions to eat later. Thaw in the refrigerator overnight and reheat to 165°F.

Per Serving (⅛ recipe): Calories: 195; Fat: 4g; Carbohydrates: 1g; Fiber: 0g; Protein: 39g; Sodium: 66mg

Roasted Sweet Potatoes *and* Cauliflower

PREP TIME: 30 minutes | COOK TIME: 40 minutes

These cauliflower steaks and potato wedges are tossed with aromatic seasonings and roasted to perfection for veggies you actually want to eat.

Nonstick cooking spray

1 teaspoon paprika

½ teaspoon sea salt

½ teaspoon freshly ground black pepper

½ teaspoon chili powder

½ teaspoon garlic powder

½ teaspoon onion powder

¼ teaspoon cayenne pepper

2 cauliflower heads, cut into ½-inch-thick steaks

¼ cup avocado oil, divided

4 cups chopped (1-inch wedges) sweet potato

DAIRY-FREE • DASH • GLUTEN-FREE • MEDITERRANEAN • SOY-FREE • VEGAN

1. Preheat the oven to 400°F. Line two baking sheets with aluminum foil and coat the foil with cooking spray.

2. In a small bowl, stir together the paprika, salt, pepper, chili powder, garlic powder, onion powder, and cayenne.

3. Drizzle the cauliflower steaks with 2 tablespoons of avocado oil, coating both sides. Sprinkle a little less than half the seasoning blend over both sides of each cauliflower steak. Place the steaks on one of the prepared baking sheets in a single layer.

4. In a large bowl, toss the sweet potato with the remaining 2 tablespoons of avocado oil and the remaining seasoning blend and spread them evenly on the second prepared baking sheet.

5. Bake the veggies for 30 to 40 minutes, or until the sweet potatoes and cauliflower are fork-tender, tossing the sweet potatoes and turning the cauliflower steaks halfway through the baking time.

6. Portion the vegetables into 8 storage containers. Refrigerate 5 containers for meals this week and freeze 3 containers for future meals.

> **NEED MORE CALORIES?** Double the amount of oil used to add healthy fat to the meal.

STORAGE TIP: Freeze the vegetables in individual portions. Thaw in the refrigerator overnight and reheat to 165°F.

INGREDIENT TIP: To cut cauliflower heads into steaks, remove the green leaves first. Cut down through the middle of the head and work your way out on each half, creating ½-inch-thick steaks. Some of them will fall apart and that's okay!

Although this recipe is indicated as gluten-free, if this is a concern for you, check the ingredient packaging to ensure all foods were processed in a completely gluten-free facility.

Per Serving (⅛ recipe): Calories: 158; Fat: 8g; Carbohydrates: 21g; Fiber: 5g; Protein: 4g; Sodium: 233mg

Steak Burrito Bowls

PREP TIME: 30 minutes | COOK TIME: 5 to 20 minutes

These sizzling and slightly spicy steak burrito bowls are filled with beans, cheese, fresh pico de gallo, guacamole, and salsa for a simple meal that works for both lunch and dinner.

1 teaspoon onion powder

1 teaspoon smoked paprika

½ teaspoon sugar

¼ teaspoon garlic powder

¼ teaspoon sea salt

⅛ teaspoon cayenne pepper

⅛ teaspoon ground chile pepper

1 pound flank steak, cut into 1-inch strips

1½ teaspoons avocado oil

4½ cups chopped romaine lettuce

1 (15-ounce) can no-salt-added black beans, drained and rinsed

¾ cup pico de gallo, drained

¾ cup shredded Mexican cheese

¾ cup salsa

⅓ cup guacamole

GLUTEN-FREE • SOY-FREE

1.   In a gallon-size freezer bag, combine the onion powder, paprika, sugar, garlic powder, salt, cayenne, and ground chile. Seal the bag and shake to mix well. Add the steak strips to the bag, reseal the bag, and shake to coat the steak well.

2.   In a cast iron skillet, heat the avocado oil over medium heat. Add the steak and cook until your desired doneness, 5 to 20 minutes (depending on how rare or well done you like steak). I recommend cooking it to 165°F if you plan to keep it for a full 5 days.

3.   In each of the 3 storage containers, arrange 1½ cups of romaine lettuce, ⅓ cup of black beans, ¼ cup of pico de gallo, and ¼ cup of cheese.

4.   In each of the 3 smaller containers, combine ¼ cup salsa and about 2 tablespoons of guacamole.

5.   Let the steak cool completely and divide it among the larger storage containers. Cover and refrigerate.

> **NEED MORE CALORIES?** Double the portion of steak, black beans, guacamole, and cheese in each bowl.

STORAGE TIP: Keep refrigerated for 3 to 5 days. You can freeze the steak separately to eat later, but the entire recipe does not freeze well.

INGREDIENT TIP: Although this recipe is indicated as gluten-free, if this is a concern for you, check the ingredient packaging to ensure all foods were processed in a completely gluten-free facility.

Per Serving (⅓ recipe): Calories: 344; Fat: 16g; Carbohydrates: 35g; Fiber: 14g; Protein: 17g; Sodium: 1,188mg

Custom Mini Quiches

PREP TIME: 30 minutes | COOK TIME: 35 minutes

Mix and match your favorite veggies and cheese to make deliciously filling mini quiches. These are great for busy mornings and making a few different types means you have variety throughout the week.

Nonstick cooking spray (optional)

¼ cup shredded Swiss cheese

½ cup chopped mushrooms

¼ cup shredded Cheddar cheese

½ cup chopped broccoli

¼ cup shredded mozzarella cheese

½ cup chopped red bell pepper

6 large eggs

2 cups liquid egg whites

6 cups grapes

DASH • GLUTEN-FREE • SOY-FREE • VEGETARIAN

1.   Preheat the oven to 375°F and line a muffin tin with silicone liners or coat it with cooking spray.

2.   In 4 muffin cups, combine 1 tablespoon of Swiss cheese and 2 tablespoons of chopped mushrooms.

3.   In 4 different muffin cups, combine 1 tablespoon of Cheddar cheese and 2 tablespoons of broccoli.

4.   In the remaining 4 muffin cups, combine 1 tablespoon of mozzarella cheese and 2 tablespoons of red bell pepper.

5.   In a medium bowl, whisk the eggs and egg whites until blended. Divide the egg mixture among the 12 muffin cups, pouring it over the cheese and veggies in each.

6. Bake for 25 to 35 minutes, or until the eggs are fully set. Remove the quiches from the muffin tin and let cool.

7. In each of the 6 storage containers, place 2 egg muffins and 1 cup of grapes. Cover and refrigerate.

NEED MORE CALORIES? Eat more egg muffins in one serving. Decrease the servings per recipe to 3 (eating 4 muffins) and make two batches so you'll have enough for the week.

STORAGE TIP: This recipe does not freeze well. Refrigerate and use within 5 to 7 days and reheat to 165°F.

INGREDIENT TIP: Although this recipe is indicated as gluten-free, if this is a concern for you, check the ingredient packaging to ensure all foods were processed in a completely gluten-free facility.

Per Serving (2 egg muffins and 1 cup grapes): Calories: 220; Fat: 8g; Carbohydrates: 18g; Fiber: 1g; Protein: 19g; Sodium: 258mg

Sheet Pan Hummus Chicken *and* Zucchini

PREP TIME: 30 minutes | **COOK TIME:** 40 minutes

Chicken topped with creamy hummus and baked to perfection is great for meal prep because the chicken stays so juicy. Paired with zucchini, this easy Mediterranean chicken dish is high in protein and low in carbs.

2 (8-ounce) boneless, skinless chicken breasts

½ cup hummus

2 medium zucchini, halved lengthwise and cut into 1-inch half-moons

1½ teaspoons avocado oil

½ teaspoon dried oregano

1 cup cooked brown rice

1 tablespoon fresh parsley, chopped

DAIRY-FREE • DASH • GLUTEN-FREE • MEDITERRANEAN • SOY-FREE

1. Preheat the oven to 425°F and line a baking sheet with parchment paper.

2. Place the chicken breasts in the center of the prepared baking sheet. Top each breast with ¼ cup of hummus. Bake for 25 minutes.

3. In a medium bowl, toss together the zucchini, avocado oil, and oregano. Arrange the zucchini in a single layer on the baking sheet around the chicken.

4. Bake for 10 to 15 minutes more, or until the chicken reaches an internal temperature of 165°F.

5. In each of the 2 storage containers, place a ½ cup of cooked brown rice, 1 chicken breast, half the zucchini, and garnish each with 1½ teaspoons of parsley.

NEED MORE CALORIES? Eat two portions of meat and top your meal with ranch dressing.

Per Serving (½ recipe): Calories: 487; Fat: 20g; Carbohydrates: 33g; Fiber: 7g; Protein: 48g; Sodium: 350mg

Peanut Butter Chocolate Energy Balls

PREP TIME: 15 minutes

These chocolate peanut butter protein balls are creamy on the outside and cake-like when you take a bite. They are filling with a delicious combination of peanut butter and chocolate that will keep cravings at bay.

1 cup rolled oats

½ cup dairy-free chocolate protein powder

½ cup natural peanut butter

⅓ cup pure maple syrup

¼ cup ground flaxseed

DAIRY-FREE • DASH • GLUTEN-FREE • MEDITERRANEAN • SOY-FREE • VEGAN

1. In a large mixing bowl, combine the oats, protein powder, peanut butter, maple syrup, and flaxseed. Stir well to mix.

2. Roll the dough into 16 (1-inch) balls, or use a cookie scoop. Refrigerate for 20 minutes before serving.

NEED MORE CALORIES? Eat more portions!

STORAGE TIP: These balls keep for 7 to 14 days in the refrigerator, or they can be frozen for up to 6 months. Thaw in the refrigerator overnight. Do not heat.

INGREDIENT TIP: Although this recipe is indicated as gluten-free, if this is a concern for you, check the ingredient packaging to ensure all foods, especially oats, were processed in a completely gluten-free facility.

Per Serving (1 ball): Calories: 106; Fat: 5g; Carbohydrates: 11g; Fiber: 1g; Protein: 5g; Sodium: 7mg

Second Five-Day Superefficient Prep Plan

This second six-recipe meal prep is designed to teach you to be super efficient with your time. By now you should be gaining some confidence in the kitchen and getting a little faster at your work, too. This week you'll cook six recipes which will keep you eating healthy for days.

SHOPPING LIST

PANTRY

- Black pepper, freshly ground
- Dill pickle relish
- Garlic powder
- Mustard, Dijon
- Oil, avocado
- Oil, olive, extra-virgin
- Onion powder
- Rice, brown
- Sea salt
- Vinegar, red wine

CANNED, BOTTLED, PACKAGED, AND PREPARED

- Beans, black, no-salt-added (1 [15-ounce] can)
- Broth, low-sodium chicken (2½ cups)
- Corn, sweet (1 [15-ounce] can)
- Enchilada sauce (1 [15-ounce] can)
- Hummus (½ cup)

FRUITS, VEGETABLES, FRESH HERBS, AND SPICES

- Avocado (1)
- Basil (1 bunch)
- Bell peppers, red (5)
- Blueberries (2½ cups)
- Carrots, baby (2 cups)
- Celery (2 stalks)
- Cilantro (2 bunches)
- Garlic (1 head)
- Grapes (5 cups)
- Lemon (1)
- Lettuce, butter (1 head)
- Mushrooms (2 cups)
- Onion, red, small (1)
- Parsley (1 bunch)
- Tomatoes, Roma (4)
- Scallions (1 bunch)
- Zucchini (10)

PROTEIN

- Chicken, rotisserie (1 [3- to 4-pound] chicken)
- Chicken thighs, boneless, skinless (2 pounds)
- Shrimp, large (1 pound)
- Tuna, water-packed (2 [5-ounce] cans)

DAIRY AND EGGS

- Cheese, feta, crumbed (1½ ounces [5 tablespoons])
- Cheese, Mexican blend, shredded (4 ounces [1 cup])
- Cheese, Parmesan rind (1)
- Cheese, Parmesan, shredded (1½ ounces [¼ cup])
- Eggs, large (10)
- Half-and-half (¼ cup)
- Yogurt, vanilla nonfat Greek (2½ cups)

	Breakfast	Lunch	Dinner	Snack
DAY 1	Stuffed Bell Peppers (page 104)	Tuna Salad Wraps (page 108)	Slow Cooker Garlic-Parmesan Chicken (page 103)	Greek Yogurt Blueberry Bites (page 109)
DAY 2	Stuffed Bell Peppers (page 104)	Tuna Salad Wraps (page 108)	Slow Cooker Garlic-Parmesan Chicken (page 103)	Greek Yogurt Blueberry Bites (page 109)
DAY 3	Stuffed Bell Peppers (page 104)	Easy Layered Enchilada Casserole (page 105)	Chimichurri Shrimp Skewers (page 107)	Greek Yogurt Blueberry Bites (page 109)
DAY 4	Stuffed Bell Peppers (page 104)	Easy Layered Enchilada Casserole (page 105)	Chimichurri Shrimp Skewers (page 107)	Greek Yogurt Blueberry Bites (page 109)
DAY 5	Stuffed Bell Peppers (page 104)	Easy Layered Enchilada Casserole (page 105)	Chimichurri Shrimp Skewers (page 107)	Greek Yogurt Blueberry Bites (page 109)

EQUIPMENT LIST

- Airtight storage containers
- Aluminum foil
- Baking sheets
- Casserole dishes: 9-by-13-inch (2) and 8-by-8-inch
- Chef's knife
- Cutting board
- Food thermometer
- Grill
- Large skillet
- Measuring cups and spoons
- Mixing bowls
- Parchment paper
- Resealable quart-size plastic bags
- Slow cooker

continued

STEP-BY-STEP GUIDE

1. Start cooking the brown rice according to the package directions for all the recipes (except **Slow Cooker Garlic-Parmesan Chicken**, page 103) or heat it in the microwave if you bought precooked.

2. Preheat the oven to 375°F.

3. Start the **Slow Cooker Garlic-Parmesan Chicken** (page 103) in the slow cooker and complete steps 1 and 2.

4. Prep the **Stuffed Bell Peppers** (page 104) and get them in the oven by completing steps 1 through 4.

5. While the stuffed peppers bake, get the **Easy Layered Enchilada Casserole** (page 105) ready to go in the oven next. Complete steps 1 through 4. You can put the enchilada casserole in the oven at the same time as the bell peppers at a higher temperature. Reduce the cooking time of the casserole by 10 minutes.

6. Get the **Chimichurri Shrimp Skewers** (page 107) ready to grill by completing steps 1 and 2.

7. When the stuffed peppers are done, remove them from the oven and finish the recipe.

8. When the enchilada casserole is done, complete the recipe and portion the servings.

9. Make the sauce for the shrimp skewers and complete the recipe.

10. Make the **Tuna Salad Wraps** (page 108).

11. Make the **Greek Yogurt Blueberry Bites** (page 109).

Slow Cooker Garlic-Parmesan Chicken

PREP TIME: 30 minutes | COOK TIME: 4 to 6 hours

Throw everything in the slow cooker and then walk away for a few hours. When you come back you'll have a cheesy, savory chicken and rice dish that is filling and comforting.

2½ cups low-sodium chicken broth

½ cup brown rice

1 Parmesan cheese rind

5 garlic cloves, minced

2 pounds boneless, skinless chicken thighs

2 cups chopped mushrooms

2 cups chopped zucchini

¼ cup chopped fresh basil

¼ cup shredded Parmesan cheese

DASH • GLUTEN-FREE • MEDITERRANEAN • SOY-FREE

1. In a slow cooker, stir together the chicken broth, brown rice, Parmesan rind, and garlic. Layer the chicken thighs on top in a single layer. Top the chicken with the mushrooms and zucchini.

2. Cover the cooker and cook on high heat for 4 to 6 hours, or until the rice is cooked and the chicken reaches an internal temperature of 165°F.

3. Remove the Parmesan rind if any is left (there might not be, which is fine) and divide the chicken, rice, and vegetables among 4 storage containers.

4. Top each with 1 tablespoon of basil and 1 tablespoon of Parmesan cheese.

NEED MORE CALORIES? Eat two portions or add more cheese!

STORAGE TIP: Freeze the meal in individual portions. Reheat from frozen or thaw in the refrigerator overnight and cook to 165°F.

Per Serving (¼ recipe): Calories: 546; Fat: 28g; Carbohydrates: 24g; Fiber: 2g; Protein: 46g; Sodium: 385mg

Stuffed Bell Peppers

PREP TIME: 15 minutes | COOK TIME: 30 minutes

Each bite of these red peppers stuffed with eggs, feta, and fresh basil will melt in your mouth. This is an antioxidant- and protein-rich meal that is simple to make.

5 large red bell peppers

10 large eggs

¼ cup half-and-half

1 teaspoon garlic powder

1 teaspoon onion powder

¼ teaspoon sea salt

¼ teaspoon freshly ground black pepper

5 tablespoons crumbled feta cheese

5 tablespoons chopped fresh basil

5 cups grapes

DASH • GLUTEN-FREE • MEDITERRANEAN • SOY-FREE • VEGETARIAN

1.   Preheat the oven to 375°F and line a 9-by-13-inch casserole dish with parchment paper.

2.   Halve the bell peppers lengthways through the stem, devein and seed them, leaving the pepper halves intact. Place the pepper halves in the prepared dish, cut-side up.

3.   In a small bowl, whisk the eggs, half-and-half, garlic powder, onion powder, salt, and pepper. Pour the eggs into the pepper halves, distributing them evenly. Sprinkle 1½ teaspoons of feta and 1½ teaspoons of basil on each.

4.   Bake for 25 to 30 minutes, or until the eggs are just set. Pack 2 bell pepper halves into each of the 5 storage containers and add 1 cup of grapes to each.

NEED MORE CALORIES? Add a side of sausage links to each meal prep container.

STORAGE TIP: Keep refrigerated for 3 to 5 days. Do not freeze.

Per Serving (1 stuffed bell pepper and 1 cup grapes): Calories: 282; Fat: 14g; Carbohydrates: 26g; Fiber: 4g; Protein: 16g; Sodium: 382mg

Easy Layered Enchilada Casserole

PREP TIME: 30 minutes | COOK TIME: 40 minutes

No rolling required for this healthy enchilada casserole topped with melted broiled cheese and filled to the brim with healthy veggies, shredded chicken, and spicy enchilada sauce.

1½ cups enchilada
  sauce, divided

1 (15-ounce) can sweet
  corn kernels, drained
  and rinsed

1 (15-ounce) can no-salt-
  added black beans,
  drained and rinsed

2 cups chopped (½-inch
  pieces) zucchini

2 cups chopped
  Roma tomato

4 cups shredded
  rotisserie chicken

1 cup shredded Mexican
  cheese blend

¼ cup chopped fresh
  cilantro

¼ cup chopped scallion,
  white and green parts

GLUTEN-FREE • MEDITERRANEAN • SOY-FREE

1. Preheat the oven to 350°F.

2. Cover the bottom of a 9-by-13-inch casserole dish with ½ cup of enchilada sauce.

3. Add the corn and beans and mix well to coat with the sauce.

4. Spread the zucchini and tomato on top of the corn and beans but do not mix.

5. Add another ½ cup of enchilada sauce and a layer of chicken.

6. Top with the remaining ½ cup of sauce and the cheese.

7. Bake for 30 to 40 minutes, or until the mixture is hot and bubbly.

continued

8.   Turn the oven to broil and broil the casserole for 3 to 5 minutes to brown. Let cool.

9.   Cut the casserole into 8 pieces and place 1 piece into each of 8 storage containers. Garnish with cilantro and scallions. Cover and refrigerate.

NEED MORE CALORIES? Eat more than one portion! You can also top with extras like guacamole and sour cream.

STORAGE TIP: Keep refrigerated for 3 to 5 days. Freeze the remaining portions in individual containers. Thaw in the refrigerator overnight and reheat to 165°F.

INGREDIENT TIP: Although this recipe is indicated as gluten-free, if this is a concern for you, check the ingredient packaging to ensure all foods were processed in a completely gluten-free facility.

Per Serving (⅛ recipe): Calories: 299; Fat: 15g; Carbohydrates: 20g; Fiber: 5g; Protein: 23g; Sodium: 900mg

Chimichurri Shrimp Skewers

PREP TIME: 30 minutes | COOK TIME: 10 minutes

These succulent shrimp skewers are grilled to perfection and drizzled with chimichurri sauce. Served over a bed of brown rice, this fragrant and bright dish is high in protein and filling.

1 pound raw large shrimp

6 cups sliced (½-inch half-moons) zucchini

1 tablespoon avocado oil

1½ teaspoons sea salt, divided

¼ teaspoon freshly ground black pepper

2 cups fresh parsley

1 cup fresh cilantro

1 scallion, green part only, chopped

1 tablespoon garlic powder

¼ cup extra-virgin olive oil

2 tablespoons red wine vinegar

1 tablespoon freshly squeezed lemon juice

1½ cups cooked brown rice

DAIRY-FREE • GLUTEN-FREE • MEDITERRANEAN • SOY-FREE

1. Preheat the grill to 400°F.

2. Add the shrimp and zucchini to skewers, alternating between one shrimp and two zucchini pieces until they are all used.

3. Brush the skewers with avocado oil and season all over with ½ teaspoon of salt and the pepper. Place the skewers on the grill and cook for 2 to 3 minutes per side until the shrimp are pink, opaque, and fully cooked.

4. In a blender, combine the parsley, cilantro, scallion, garlic powder, olive oil, vinegar, lemon juice, and remaining 1 teaspoon of salt. Process until smooth. Drizzle the chimichurri sauce over the skewers.

5. In each of the 3 storage containers, place ½ cup of brown rice. Divide the shrimp and zucchini among the containers.

NEED MORE CALORIES? Double the portion of rice and shrimp.

INGREDIENT TIP: Although this recipe is indicated as gluten-free, if this is a concern for you, check the ingredient packaging to ensure all foods, especially oats, were processed in a completely gluten-free facility.

Per Serving (⅓ recipe): Calories: 491; Fat: 25g; Carbohydrates: 36g; Fiber: 7g; Protein: 36g; Sodium: 976mg

Tuna Salad Wraps

PREP TIME: 15 minutes

This tuna salad is creamy with bits of dill pickle, celery, and onion to add crunch. This recipe is healthier and more weight-loss friendly than traditional tuna salad because it swaps mashed avocado and hummus for traditional mayonnaise.

1 avocado, halved, pitted, and peeled

2 (5-ounce) cans low-sodium water-packed solid white albacore tuna, drained

½ cup hummus

½ cup chopped celery

¼ cup dill pickle relish

2 tablespoons chopped red onion

2 tablespoons Dijon mustard

¼ teaspoon freshly ground black pepper

Sea salt

4 butter lettuce leaves

2 cups baby carrots

DAIRY-FREE • MEDITERRANEAN • SOY-FREE

1.   In a medium bowl, using a fork, mash the avocado. Add the tuna, hummus, celery, relish, red onion, mustard, and pepper. Mix well. Season with salt. Divide the tuna salad between 2 (divided, if you have them) storage containers.

2.   In 2 separate containers, or the divided containers, place 2 lettuce leaves, and 1 cup of baby carrots.

NEED MORE CALORIES? Eat double portions.

STORAGE TIP: Keep refrigerated for up to 3 days. This recipe is not freezer friendly.

Per Serving (½ recipe): Calories: 515; Fat: 26g; Carbohydrates: 44g; Fiber: 16g; Protein: 25g; Sodium: 1,050mg

SERVES 5

Greek Yogurt Blueberry Bites

PREP TIME: 20 minutes

These blueberries are coated in a sweet creamy layer of Greek yogurt for a flavor sensation. Eat these sweet frozen treats straight from the freezer for a snack or a healthy dessert.

2½ cups fresh blueberries

2½ cups vanilla nonfat Greek yogurt

DASH • GLUTEN-FREE • MEDITERRANEAN • SOY-FREE • VEGETARIAN

1. Line a baking sheet with wax paper or parchment paper.

2. In a medium bowl, stir together the blueberries and yogurt so each berry is coated. Scoop out the blueberries individually and place them on the prepared baking sheet. Freeze for at least 4 hours.

3. Into each of the 5 resealable plastic bags, place ½ cup of frozen blueberries. Seal the bags and freeze until you are ready to eat.

NEED MORE CALORIES? Roll the berries in full-fat yogurt.

INGREDIENT TIP: Although this recipe is indicated as gluten-free, if this is a concern for you, check the ingredient packaging to ensure all foods were processed in a completely gluten-free facility.

Per Serving (½ cup): Calories: 138; Fat: 0g; Carbohydrates: 25g; Fiber: 2g; Protein: 21g; Sodium: 40mg

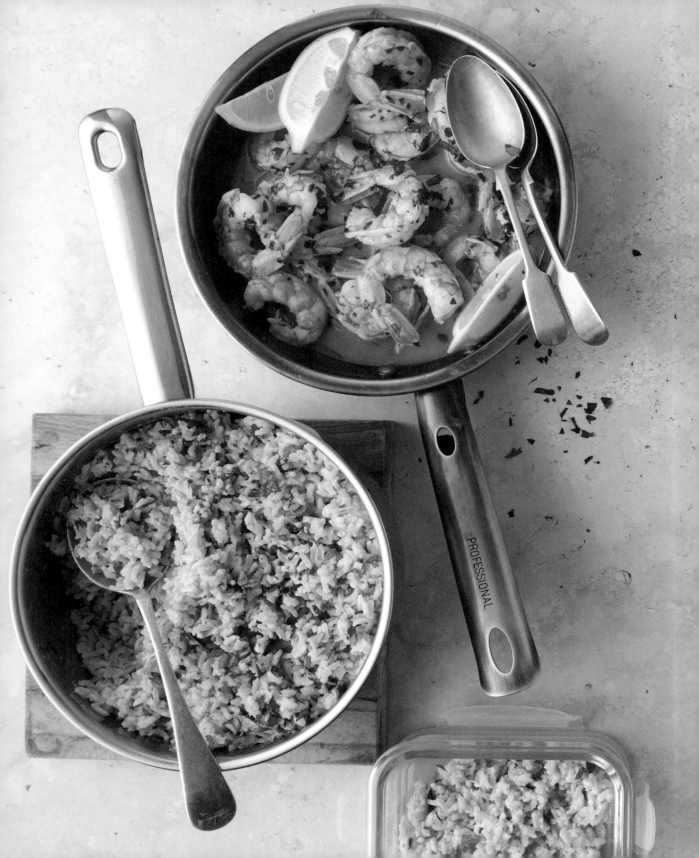

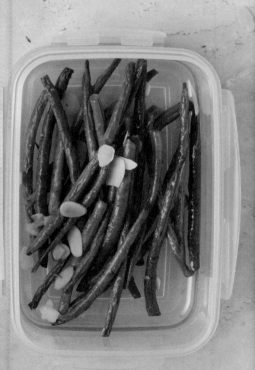
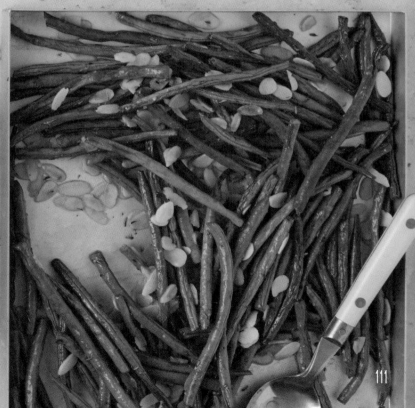

PART THREE

BATCH-FRIENDLY

Recipes

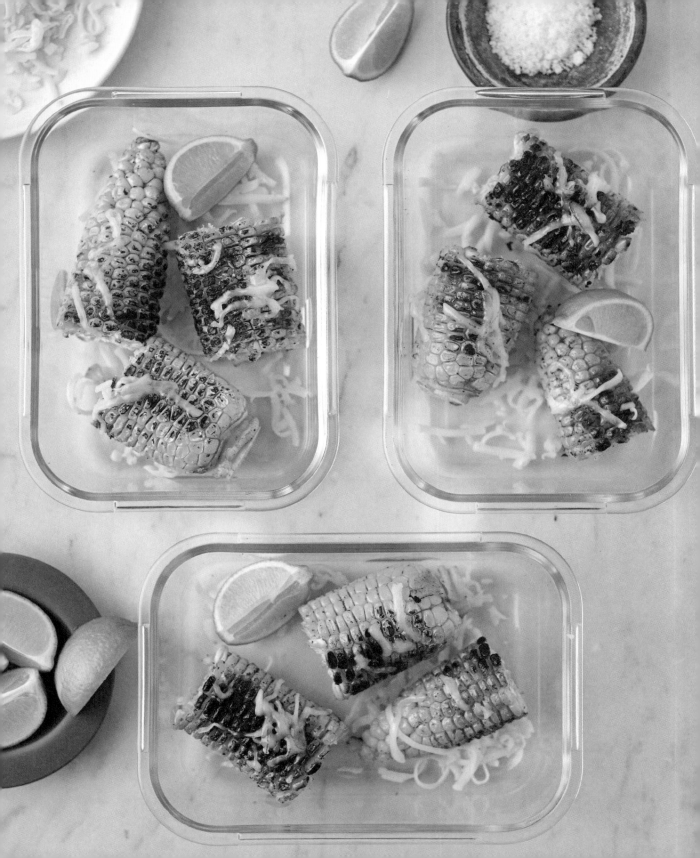

CHAPTER SEVEN

Healthy Carb Recipes

Cinnamon-Roasted Sweet Potatoes 114

Coconut-Lime Brown Rice 115

Roasted Garlic-Parmesan Quinoa 116

Customizable Protein Steel Cut Oatmeal Cups 117

Tangy and Spicy Perfect Plantains 119

Mixed Herb Smashed Red Potatoes 120

Parmesan Polenta Rounds 122

Grilled Chili-Lime Fiesta Corn 123

Caramelized Butternut Squash and Farro Salad 124

Muffin Tin Mini Lentil Loaves 126

《 Grilled Chili-Lime Fiesta Corn (page 123)

Cinnamon-Roasted Sweet Potatoes

PREP TIME: 5 minutes | COOK TIME: 25 minutes

Sweet potatoes contain fewer calories and carbs per ounce and are higher in fiber and vitamin A than white potatoes. These cinnamon sweet potatoes are roasted until caramelized on the outside and tender on the inside. These potatoes work as a breakfast potato with hard-boiled eggs or turkey sausage. They're also delicious for dinner paired with savory recipes like chicken or turkey.

Nonstick cooking spray

2 large sweet potatoes, cut into 1-inch cubes (4 cups chopped sweet potato)

1 tablespoon coconut oil

1 tablespoon ground cinnamon

DAIRY-FREE • DASH • GLUTEN-FREE • MEDITERRANEAN • SOY-FREE • VEGAN

1. Preheat the oven to 400°F. Line a baking sheet with parchment paper and coat it with cooking spray.

2. In a medium bowl, toss the sweet potatoes, coconut oil, and cinnamon to coat. Evenly spread the sweet potatoes onto the prepared baking sheet.

3. Bake for 25 minutes until fork-tender.

NEED MORE CALORIES? Double this recipe or toss with slivered almonds during the last 10 to 15 minutes of baking.

STORAGE TIP: Freeze the sweet potatoes in a single batch or as individual portions. Thaw in the microwave, or in the refrigerator overnight, and reheat to 165°F.

INGREDIENT TIP: Although this recipe is indicated as gluten-free, if this is a concern for you, check the ingredient packaging to ensure all foods were processed in a completely gluten-free facility.

Per Serving (⅛ recipe): Calories: 74; Fat: 2g; Carbohydrates: 14g; Fiber: 3g; Protein: 1g; Sodium: 37mg

Coconut-Lime Brown Rice

PREP TIME: 5 minutes | COOK TIME: 40 minutes

Creamy coconut-lime brown rice has a slightly nutty texture and a fresh burst of Caribbean flavors—coconut, lime, and cilantro. This rice makes a great side for rotisserie chicken, shredded chicken, or baked shrimp.

4 cups coconut milk (from a carton)

2 cups brown rice

Juice of 2 limes

Grated zest of 2 limes

¼ cup chopped fresh cilantro

Sea salt

DAIRY-FREE • DASH • GLUTEN-FREE • MEDITERRANEAN • SOY-FREE • VEGAN

1.　In a large pot over high heat, bring the coconut milk to a boil. Add the brown rice, reduce the heat to maintain a simmer, and cover the pot. Cook for 30 to 40 minutes until the liquid is absorbed and the rice is tender.

2.　Stir in the lime juice, lime zest, and cilantro. Season with salt.

NEED MORE CALORIES? Make a double batch and double your portion, or stir in some coconut cream for a creamier texture and more fat.

STORAGE TIP: Freeze the rice in a single batch or in individual portions. Thaw in the microwave, or in the refrigerator overnight, and reheat to 165°F.

INGREDIENT TIP: Although this recipe is indicated as gluten-free, if this is a concern for you, check the ingredient packaging to ensure all foods, especially oats, were processed in a completely gluten-free facility.

Per Serving (½ cup): Calories: 212; Fat: 4g; Carbohydrates: 40g; Fiber: 2g; Protein: 4g; Sodium: 21mg

Roasted Garlic-Parmesan Quinoa

PREP TIME: 5 minutes | COOK TIME: 30 minutes

Quinoa is one of the whole grains with the highest amount of protein and fiber, making it more filling than other grains. This fluffy quinoa dish has creamy roasted garlic stirred into it and is topped with Parmesan cheese. It pairs well with roasted or steamed veggies.

1 garlic head

1 teaspoon avocado oil

Sea salt

4 cups water

2 cups quinoa, rinsed

½ cup shredded
   Parmesan cheese

DASH • GLUTEN-FREE • MEDITERRANEAN • SOY-FREE • VEGETARIAN

1. Preheat the oven to 400°F.

2. Cut the top off the garlic head to expose the cloves. Drizzle the avocado oil on top and sprinkle with sea salt. Wrap the garlic in aluminum foil and place it on a baking sheet.

3. Bake for 30 minutes until brown and tender.

4. While the garlic roasts, in a large pot with a lid over high heat, combine the water and quinoa and bring to a boil. Reduce the heat to maintain a simmer, cover the pot, and cook for 15 minutes until all the liquid is absorbed and the quinoa is fluffy.

5. Squeeze 7 to 10 roasted garlic cloves from their skins (more if you love garlic; less if you don't) and stir them into the quinoa. Top with the Parmesan cheese.

NEED MORE CALORIES? Eat two portions or stir in some extra-virgin olive oil for more calories.

STORAGE TIP: Freeze the quinoa in a single batch or in individual portions. Thaw in the microwave, or in the refrigerator overnight, and reheat to 165°F. To freeze leftover roasted garlic, remove the cloves from their skins and then freeze in an airtight container.

Per Serving (⅙ recipe): Calories: 253; Fat: 7g; Carbohydrates: 37g; Fiber: 4g; Protein: 11g; Sodium: 93mg

Customizable Protein Steel Cut Oatmeal Cups

PREP TIME: 10 minutes | COOK TIME: 15 minutes

Steel cut oatmeal is a heartier, nuttier type of oatmeal that has a delightfully chewy texture. Although all oats are good for you, steel cut oats have slightly fewer calories and cause a steadier blood sugar response compared to rolled oats.

Nonstick cooking spray

6 cups water, plus more as needed

2 cups quick cooking steel cut oats

1 cup protein powder

2 tablespoons ground cinnamon

1 teaspoon vanilla extract

8 drops stevia (optional)

2 cups fresh blueberries

⅓ cup slivered almonds

DAIRY-FREE • DASH • GLUTEN-FREE • MEDITERRANEAN • SOY-FREE • VEGAN

1. Coat two silicone muffin tins with cooking spray.

2. In a large pot over high heat, bring the water to a boil. Add the oats and cook for 7 to 9 minutes, or until the oats are tender and the liquid is absorbed.

3. Stir in the protein powder, cinnamon, vanilla, and stevia (if using). Add more water as needed to keep the desired consistency.

4. Place ⅓ cup of oatmeal into each prepared muffin cup. Top each with blueberries and almonds. Place the tin in the freezer until the oatmeal is frozen.

continued

5.   Remove the oatmeal cups and transfer them to a plastic freezer bag. Seal and freeze until needed, or up to 6 months.

6.   To reheat, place the oatmeal cups in a wide-mouth Mason jar and let them thaw in the refrigerator overnight. Reheat in the microwave for about 1 minute, or microwave them from frozen for about 2 minutes. For a creamier dish, add ¼ cup milk or water while reheating.

NEED MORE CALORIES? Eat 2 servings or stir in some almond butter or peanut butter for added healthy fat and protein. Incorporate the mix-ins before freezing or once the oatmeal is hot.

INGREDIENT TIP: Use any combination of fruit and nut you like. Shredded apple and walnuts are delicious.

Although this recipe is indicated as gluten-free, if this is a concern for you, check the ingredient packaging to ensure all foods, especially oats, were processed in a completely gluten-free facility.

Per Serving (1 oat "muffin"): Calories: 83; Fat: 2g; Carbohydrates: 13g; Fiber: 2g; Protein: 5g; Sodium: 7mg

Tangy *and* Spicy Perfect Plantains

PREP TIME: 10 minutes | **COOK TIME:** 10 minutes

Ripe plantains have a tangy sweet flavor and are yellow with black spots. They are a rich source of fiber, vitamins A, B$_6$, and C as well as the minerals magnesium and potassium. These plantains are lightly fried to a crisp and are tangy with a hint of heat that pairs well with chicken seasoned with Caribbean spices or seafood. They're even delicious for breakfast.

3 large ripe plantains, cut into ¼-inch-thick slices

¼ teaspoon sea salt, plus more for seasoning

¼ teaspoon ground cinnamon

⅛ teaspoon cayenne pepper

2 tablespoons avocado oil

DAIRY-FREE • DASH • GLUTEN-FREE • MEDITERRANEAN • SOY-FREE • VEGAN

1. Sprinkle the plantain slices with sea salt, cinnamon, and cayenne.

2. In a large skillet, heat the avocado oil over medium heat.

3. Working in batches as needed, add the plantain slices and cook for 1 to 2 minutes per side until golden brown and crispy.

4. Using tongs, transfer the plantain slices to paper towels to drain any residual oil. Taste and season with salt, as needed.

NEED MORE CALORIES? Eat more than one portion; this recipe can easily be doubled using two skillets at once or cooking more batches.

STORAGE TIP: Freeze the plantain slices in a single batch or in individual portions, or refrigerate for up to 5 days. Thaw in the microwave, or in the refrigerator overnight, and reheat to 165°F.

Per Serving (½ cup): Calories: 206; Fat: 5g; Carbohydrates: 43g; Fiber: 2g; Protein: 2g; Sodium: 104mg

Mixed Herb Smashed Red Potatoes

PREP TIME: 10 minutes | **COOK TIME:** 35 minutes

These potatoes are boiled, smashed, drizzled with herbs and oil, and roasted to crispy golden-brown perfection.

2 pounds red potatoes

1 bay leaf

Nonstick cooking spray

3 tablespoons avocado oil

1 teaspoon dried parsley

1 teaspoon garlic powder

1 teaspoon dried oregano

¼ teaspoon sea salt

DAIRY-FREE • DASH • GLUTEN-FREE • MEDITERRANEAN • SOY-FREE • VEGAN

1. In a large pot, combine the potatoes with enough water to cover. Add the bay leaf. Place the pot over high heat and bring the water to a boil. Cook for 10 to 15 minutes until the potatoes are fork-tender but not falling apart. Remove and discard the bay leaf. Drain the potatoes and set aside to cool for 10 minutes.

2. Preheat the oven to 425°F. Line a baking sheet with parchment paper and coat it with cooking spray. (Depending on the size of your potatoes, you may need two baking sheets.)

3. In a small bowl, stir together the avocado oil, parsley, garlic powder, oregano, and salt.

4. Place the potatoes on the prepared baking sheet and, using a potato masher or fork, press down to slightly smash the potatoes. Brush the herbed oil onto the potatoes, covering the whole potato.

5. Bake for 15 to 20 minutes, or until they start to crisp and are golden brown. (If using two baking sheets, switch the sheets to alternate racks and turn them front to back halfway through the cooking time.)

NEED MORE CALORIES? Top the potatoes with a flavorful cheese like Gouda, Parmesan, or Cheddar. Once the potatoes finish baking, sprinkle them with 3 to 4 ounces of shredded cheese and broil for 1 to 2 minutes.

STORAGE TIP: This recipe doesn't freeze well. The potatoes lose a lot of their texture if you freeze them. Keep refrigerated and use within 5 to 7 days.

COOKING TIP: If you reheat these in the microwave, they will lose some of their crispiness but will still be delicious. If you are able, reheat them in the toaster oven so they stay crispy.

INGREDIENT TIP: Although this recipe is indicated as gluten-free, if this is a concern for you, check the ingredient packaging to ensure all foods were processed in a completely gluten-free facility.

Per Serving (⅕ recipe): Calories: 209; Fat: 8g; Carbohydrates: 32g; Fiber: 3g; Protein: 4g; Sodium: 118mg

Parmesan Polenta Rounds

PREP TIME: 10 minutes | COOK TIME: 40 minutes

Polenta, often known as grits, is typically a creamy dish, but this recipe utilizes polenta in solid form to create a deliciously crispy cheesy side dish. The polenta rounds pair well with baked tofu, roasted edamame, roasted chicken, or anything that goes with marinara sauce.

Nonstick cooking spray

1 (17.6-ounce) tube polenta, cut into ¼-inch-thick rounds

½ teaspoon garlic powder

⅛ teaspoon freshly ground black pepper

½ cup marinara sauce

½ cup shredded or grated Parmesan cheese

DASH • GLUTEN-FREE • MEDITERRANEAN • SOY-FREE • VEGETARIAN

1. Preheat the oven to 400°F. Line a baking sheet with aluminum foil and coat it with cooking spray.

2. Place the polenta rounds on the prepared baking sheet. Season with garlic powder and pepper.

3. Bake for 20 minutes.

4. Top each round with ½ teaspoon of marinara sauce and 1 teaspoon of Parmesan cheese.

5. Bake for 20 minutes more. If desired, adjust the oven to broil and broil for 1 to 2 minutes to further crisp the tops of the polenta rounds.

NEED MORE CALORIES? Eat double portions.

STORAGE TIP: Freeze the rounds in a single batch or in individual portions. Thaw in the microwave, or in the refrigerator overnight, and reheat to 165°F in the microwave for a quick reheat, or, to retain crispness, in a toaster oven. Serve with leftover marinara sauce.

Per Serving (about 1½ ounces): Calories: 194; Fat: 1g; Carbohydrates: 40g; Fiber: 1g; Protein: 6g; Sodium: 72mg

Grilled Chili-Lime Fiesta Corn

PREP TIME: 5 minutes | **COOK TIME:** 20 minutes

The grill is great for meal prep. Every crunchy bite of this corn will be slightly limey and salty with a bit of heat and creamy Oaxaca cheese.

1½ tablespoons grated
   lime zest

1 teaspoon chili powder

½ teaspoon sea salt

5 ears sweet corn, husked

2 tablespoons avocado oil

1 lime, cut into wedges

¼ cup Oaxaca cheese

DASH • GLUTEN-FREE • MEDITERRANEAN • SOY-FREE • VEGETARIAN

1. Preheat the grill to 450°F.

2. In a small bowl, combine the zest, chili powder, and salt.

3. Brush each piece of corn with avocado oil and sprinkle with the seasoning blend. Wrap each ear in aluminum foil.

4. Place the wrapped corn on the grill and cook for 20 minutes until the corn is tender and charred, flipping them every 5 minutes so you get even charring.

5. Serve with a lime wedge for squeezing and sprinkle of Oaxaca cheese, about 1 scant tablespoon per ear.

> **NEED MORE CALORIES?** Cut the kernels off the ears and mix with twice the amount of cheese. Add canned black beans, rinsed and drained, for more starch and some added protein.

STORAGE TIP: To freeze, cut the kernels off the cobs and freeze in individual portions. After thawing, reheat to 165°F.

INGREDIENT TIP: Although this recipe is indicated as gluten-free, check the ingredient packaging to ensure all foods were processed in a completely gluten-free facility.

Per Serving (1 ear): Calories: 156; Fat: 8g; Carbohydrates: 19g; Fiber: 1g; Protein: 4g; Sodium: 272mg

Caramelized Butternut Squash *and* Farro Salad

PREP TIME: 10 minutes | COOK TIME: 40 minutes

Caramelized butternut squash is tossed with warm, chewy farro, tart dried cranberries, and crunchy pumpkin seeds in this seasonal favorite. Finish the salad with a drizzle of balsamic glaze for a sweet accent. Pair this with Lemon-Pepper Dill Salmon Foil Packets (page 146) or any other protein and veggie. Because this dish has a decent amount of protein, you can also use it as both a protein and carb meal prep dish.

1 pound butternut
   squash cubes

1 tablespoon avocado oil

1 tablespoon pure
   maple syrup

¼ teaspoon sea salt

1 cup farro, rinsed

3 cups water

¼ cup dried unsweetened
   cranberries

¼ cup pumpkin seeds

3 tablespoons
   balsamic glaze

DAIRY-FREE • DASH • GLUTEN-FREE • MEDITERRANEAN • SOY-FREE • VEGAN

1. Preheat the oven to 400°F and line a baking sheet with parchment paper.

2. Spread the butternut squash cubes in a single layer on the prepared baking sheet.

3. In a small bowl, stir together the avocado oil, maple syrup, and salt. Pour the mixture over the squash and toss to coat.

4. Bake for 20 minutes or until the squash is fork-tender.

5. Meanwhile, in a medium pot over high heat, combine the farro and water and bring to a boil. Reduce the heat to medium-low and simmer, uncovered, for 30 minutes. Drain off any excess liquid and transfer the farro to a large bowl.

6. Add the butternut squash, cranberries, and pumpkin seeds. Gently stir to mix and drizzle with balsamic glaze. Serve hot or cold.

NEED MORE CALORIES? Double the amount of cranberries and pumpkin seeds for extra carbs and fat.

STORAGE TIP: Freeze this salad in a single batch or in individual portions. Thaw in the microwave, or in the refrigerator overnight, and reheat to 165°F.

INGREDIENT TIP: Although this recipe is indicated as gluten-free, if this is a concern for you, check the ingredient packaging to ensure all foods, especially oats, were processed in a completely gluten-free facility.

Per Serving: (about ¾ cup): Calories: 221; Fat: 5g; Carbohydrates: 38g; Fiber: 4g; Protein: 8g; Sodium: 108mg

Muffin Tin Mini Lentil Loaves

PREP TIME: 15 minutes | COOK TIME: 40 minutes

These mini lentil loaves are so bursting with crunchy veggies and flavor that you'd never guess they didn't have any meat. Lentils are high in protein and fiber and make a delicious meat substitute for meatless Monday. Although this recipe is in the healthy carbohydrates section, it also provides a decent amount of carbohydrates and counts for both your protein and carb meal prep.

6 tablespoons ground
   flaxseed meal

¾ cup water

Nonstick cooking spray

2 tablespoons avocado oil

1 white onion, chopped

4 garlic cloves, minced

1 cup chopped celery

4 cups cooked lentils

2 cups quick cooking oats

1 cup chickpea flour

¼ cup tomato paste

¼ cup low-sodium
   soy sauce

2 tablespoons
   dried oregano

1 teaspoon ground
   chipotle pepper

1 teaspoon sea salt

1 teaspoon freshly ground
   black pepper

½ cup low-sugar
   barbecue sauce

DAIRY-FREE • MEDITERRANEAN • VEGAN

1. In a small bowl, stir together the flaxseed meal and water. Refrigerate the mixture for at least 10 minutes.

2. Preheat the oven to 350°F and lightly coat two silicone muffin tins with cooking spray.

3. In a skillet, heat the avocado oil over medium heat. Add the onion and garlic and cook for about 1 minute until the onion is translucent. Add the celery. Sauté for 3 to 5 minutes until soft.

4. Transfer half the vegetables to a food processor and add half each of the lentils, oats, flour, tomato paste, soy sauce, oregano, chipotle pepper, salt, black pepper, and soaked flax-seed meal. Pulse 10 to 12 times. Scrape down the bowl and pulse again until the mixture is well combined but still has visible lentils (you don't want a purée).

5. Fill the prepared muffin tins with the mixture, about ⅓ cup for each well.

6. Repeat steps 4 and 5 with the remaining half of the ingredients.

7. Brush each muffin top with barbecue sauce.

8. Bake for 30 minutes until browned and firm.

NEED MORE CALORIES? Eat more mini lentil loaves!

STORAGE TIP: Freeze the loaves in a single batch or in individual portions. Thaw in the microwave, or in the refrigerator overnight, and reheat to 165°F.

INGREDIENT TIP: To make this recipe gluten-free and soy-free, use coconut aminos instead of the soy sauce.

Per Serving (3 muffins): Calories: 373; Fat: 8g; Carbohydrates: 57g; Fiber: 11g; Protein: 20g; Sodium: 605mg

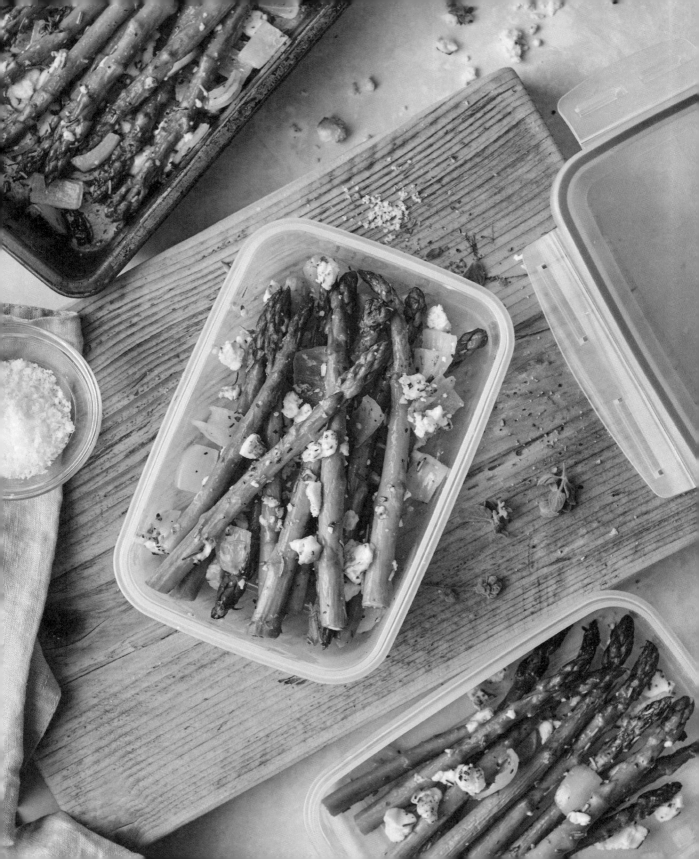

CHAPTER EIGHT

Delicious and Healthy Veggies

Herb-Roasted Asparagus and Feta 130

Crunchy Roasted Green Beans with Slivered Almonds 131

Glazed Slow Cooker Carrots 132

Crispy Roasted Greek Vegetable Medley 133

Crispy Roasted Garlicky Brussels Sprouts 135

Foil Packet Parmesan Squash 136

Spaghetti Squash 137

Marinated Cucumber and Tomato Salad 139

Teriyaki Eggplant 140

Chinese Five-Spice Bok Choy 141

《 Herb-Roasted Asparagus and Feta (page 130)

Herb-Roasted Asparagus *and* Feta

PREP TIME: 10 minutes | COOK TIME: 35 minutes

Asparagus is low in calories and high in antioxidants, and studies show it can also help lower blood pressure. These asparagus spears are tossed with seasonings, onions, and feta cheese then roasted until tender.

1½ pounds asparagus spears, woody ends trimmed

½ yellow onion, chopped into chunks

1½ teaspoons avocado oil

½ teaspoon dried oregano

½ teaspoon dried crushed rosemary

½ teaspoon garlic powder

¼ teaspoon freshly ground black pepper

½ cup crumbled feta cheese

DASH • GLUTEN-FREE • MEDITERRANEAN • SOY-FREE • VEGETARIAN

1. Preheat the oven to 400°F.

2. In an 8-by-8-inch baking dish, toss the asparagus, onion, avocado oil, oregano, rosemary, garlic powder, and pepper to coat. Sprinkle the feta on top.

3. Bake for 30 to 35 minutes, tossing the asparagus halfway through the baking time, until the asparagus is fork-tender.

NEED MORE CALORIES? Toss the asparagus with twice as much avocado oil and feta cheese.

STORAGE TIP: Freeze the asparagus in a single batch or in individual portions. Thaw in the microwave, or in the refrigerator overnight, and reheat to 165°F.

INGREDIENT TIP: Although this recipe is indicated as gluten-free, if this is a concern for you, check the ingredient packaging to ensure all foods were processed in a completely gluten-free facility.

Per Serving (¼ recipe): Calories: 105; Fat: 6g; Carbohydrates: 9g; Fiber: 4g; Protein: 7g; Sodium: 217mg

Crunchy Roasted Green Beans
with Slivered Almonds

PREP TIME: 10 minutes | COOK TIME: 45 minutes to 1 hour

Green beans are rich in vitamin K, which is needed for strong bones. These green beans are roasted with crunchy, salty almonds for the perfect nutty-fresh combination. The almonds will fall to the bottom of the dish and roast. Make sure you scoop them from the bottom and add a spoonful to every portion when serving.

24 ounces haricot vert green beans, trimmed

2 tablespoons avocado oil

1 teaspoon dried crushed thyme

1 teaspoon garlic sea salt

¼ cup raw slivered almonds

DAIRY-FREE • DASH • GLUTEN-FREE • MEDITERRANEAN • SOY-FREE • VEGAN

---

1.   Preheat the oven to 350°F.

2.   In a 9-by-13-inch baking dish, toss the green beans, avocado oil, thyme, garlic salt, and almonds to coat.

3.   Bake for 45 to 60 minutes, stirring once halfway through the cooking time, until the green beans are fork-tender and slightly browned.

> **NEED MORE CALORIES?** Add another tablespoon of avocado oil and add another ¼ cup of slivered almonds to the recipe.

STORAGE TIP: Freeze the green beans in a single batch or in individual portions. Thaw in the microwave, or in the refrigerator overnight, and reheat to 165°F.

Per Serving (⅙ recipe): Calories: 84; Fat: 7g; Carbohydrates: 4g; Fiber: 2g; Protein: 2g; Sodium: 111mg

Glazed Slow Cooker Carrots

PREP TIME: 10 minutes | **COOK TIME:** 4 hours, 20 minutes

Carrots are low in calories and naturally sweet. This recipe slow cooks the carrots until very tender and adds a buttery sugar glaze with notes of cinnamon and nutmeg.

3 tablespoons
melted butter

3 tablespoons light
brown sugar

½ teaspoon ground
cinnamon

¼ teaspoon ground nutmeg

2 pounds baby carrots,
or regular carrots cut
into coins

DASH • GLUTEN-FREE • MEDITERRANEAN • SOY-FREE •
VEGETARIAN

1.   In a small bowl, whisk the melted butter, brown sugar, cinnamon, and nutmeg.

2.   In the slow cooker, combine the carrots and the butter mixture. Toss to coat the carrots evenly.

3.   Cover the cooker and cook on high heat for 3 to 4 hours, or until the carrots are fork-tender.

4.   Remove the lid and cook for 15 to 20 minutes more to thicken the sauce into a glaze.

> **NEED MORE CALORIES?** Double the amount of butter and sugar.

STORAGE TIP: Freeze the carrots in a single batch or in individual portions. Thaw in the microwave, or in the refrigerator overnight, and reheat to 165°F.

INGREDIENT TIP: Make this recipe dairy-free by using a vegan butter substitute or coconut oil instead of the dairy butter.

Although this recipe is indicated as gluten-free, if this is a concern for you, check the ingredient packaging to ensure all foods were processed in a completely gluten-free facility.

Per Serving (¼ recipe): Calories: 212; Fat: 9g; Carbohydrates: 32g; Fiber: 8g; Protein: 0g; Sodium: 262mg

Crispy Roasted Greek Vegetable Medley

PREP TIME: 15 minutes | COOK TIME: 45 minutes

The more colors, the more nutrients—and this colorful dish packs both flavor and nutrients. Zucchini and eggplants are high in antioxidants, while bell peppers are rich in vitamin C. This dish could, technically, be eaten raw but roasting brings out the depth of the vegetables' flavors for a richer taste in every bite.

Nonstick cooking spray

2 zucchini, cut into ½-inch half-moons

1 red bell pepper, cut into 1-inch pieces

1 yellow bell pepper, cut into 1-inch pieces

1 eggplant, cut into 1-inch pieces

½ cup diced (¼ inch) red onion

2 tablespoons avocado oil

2 teaspoons salt-free Italian seasoning

½ teaspoon dried mint

¼ teaspoon freshly ground black pepper

¼ teaspoon sea salt

1 tablespoon balsamic glaze

DAIRY-FREE • DASH • GLUTEN-FREE • MEDITERRANEAN • SOY-FREE • VEGAN

1. Preheat the oven to 425°F. Line two baking sheets with aluminum foil and lightly coat them with cooking spray.

2. In a large bowl, toss together the zucchini, red and yellow bell peppers, eggplant, red onion, avocado oil, Italian seasoning, mint, pepper, and salt to coat. Divide the vegetables between the prepared baking sheets.

3. Bake for 30 to 45 minutes, or until the vegetables are slightly crisp and fork-tender, switching racks halfway through the baking time and turning the sheet front to back.

4. Drizzle the balsamic glaze over the vegetables and serve.

NEED MORE CALORIES? Toss the roasted veggies with feta cheese or slivered almonds once out of the oven.

continued

STORAGE TIP: Freeze the roasted veggies in a single batch or in individual portions. Thaw in the microwave, or in the refrigerator overnight, and reheat to 165°F.

INGREDIENT TIP: Although this recipe is indicated as gluten-free, if this is a concern for you, check the ingredient packaging to ensure all foods were processed in a completely gluten-free facility.

Per Serving (¼ recipe): Calories: 144; Fat: 8g; Carbohydrates: 18g; Fiber: 6g; Protein: 3g; Sodium: 160mg

Crispy Roasted Garlicky Brussels Sprouts

PREP TIME: 10 minutes | COOK TIME: 25 minutes

Caraway seeds are typically found in rye bread and are known to have stomach-settling properties, including anti-gas, which is why we pair them with Brussels sprouts in this recipe.

2 pounds petite Brussels sprouts, trimmed and halved

2 tablespoons avocado oil

1 tablespoon garlic powder

1 teaspoon caraway seeds (optional)

¼ teaspoon sea salt

DAIRY-FREE • DASH • GLUTEN-FREE • MEDITERRANEAN • SOY-FREE • VEGAN

1. Preheat the oven to 400°F and line a baking sheet with heavy-duty aluminum foil.

2. In a medium bowl, toss together the Brussels sprouts, avocado oil, garlic powder, caraway seeds (if using), and salt to coat. Spread the Brussels sprouts evenly on the prepared baking sheet.

3. Bake for 20 to 25 minutes until crispy and fork-tender.

NEED MORE CALORIES? Sprinkle the roasted Brussels sprouts with Parmesan cheese.

STORAGE TIP: Freeze the Brussels sprouts in a single batch or in individual portions. Thaw in the microwave, or in the refrigerator overnight, and reheat to 165°F. If you freeze these, the Brussels sprouts will not be crispy when you eat them, but they will still be garlicky and delicious!

INGREDIENT TIP: Although this recipe is indicated as gluten-free, if this is a concern for you, check the ingredient packaging to ensure all foods were processed in a completely gluten-free facility.

Per Serving (¼ recipe): Calories: 119; Fat: 7g; Carbohydrates: 12g; Fiber: 5g; Protein: 4g; Sodium: 177mg

Foil Packet Parmesan Squash

PREP TIME: 10 minutes | **COOK TIME:** 15 minutes

A crispy cheese topping covers layers of roasted summer squash in this simple dish.

2 medium zucchini, cut into ½-inch-thick half-moons

2 medium yellow squash, cut into ½-inch-thick half-moons

2 tablespoons avocado oil

¼ cup grated Parmesan cheese

½ teaspoon dried oregano

1 tablespoon chopped fresh basil

DASH • GLUTEN-FREE • MEDITERRANEAN • SOY-FREE • VEGETARIAN

1. Preheat the grill, or the oven, to 450°F. Cut two 18-by-18-inch pieces of heavy-duty aluminum foil.

2. In a large bowl, toss the zucchini, squash, avocado oil, Parmesan cheese, and oregano to coat. Place half the zucchini on each piece of foil and fold all sides up and over to seal the packet.

3. Place the packets on the grill and cook 10 to 15 minutes until the zucchini is tender.

4. Garnish the grilled zucchini with fresh basil before serving.

> **NEED MORE CALORIES?** Toss with additional grated or shredded Parmesan cheese before eating.

STORAGE TIP: This recipe is not freezer friendly. Keep refrigerated for up to 5 days.

INGREDIENT TIP: Although this recipe is indicated as gluten-free, if this is a concern for you, check the ingredient packaging to ensure all foods were processed in a completely gluten-free facility.

Per Serving (¼ recipe): Calories: 123; Fat: 10g; Carbohydrates: 6g; Fiber: 2g; Protein: 5g; Sodium: 61mg

Spaghetti Squash

PREP TIME: 5 minutes | COOK TIME: 10 minutes to 4 hours, depending on cooking method

Cover this spaghetti squash with your favorite pasta sauce—you can use even the high-calorie ones like pesto or Alfredo and still lose weight. Spaghetti squash contains only 30 calories and 7 grams of carbs per cup, compared to 190 calories and 32 grams of carbohydrates for 1 cup of cooked pasta. When prepared correctly—and I show you three ways to do that here—the spaghetti squash should not be mushy. It should be tender enough to eat but with a slight crunch.

1 medium spaghetti squash

DAIRY-FREE • DASH • GLUTEN-FREE • MEDITERRANEAN • SOY-FREE • VEGAN

MICROWAVE METHOD

1.   Using a sharp knife, cut slits in the squash in a dash pattern around the length of the spaghetti squash (as if you were going to halve it lengthwise). Place it in a microwave-safe dish and microwave on high power for 7 to 9 minutes until the squash dents when pushed without mushing (then it's overdone).

2.   Cut the squash in half along the slits and, using kitchen shears, cut out the seeds and threads.

3.   Using a fork, work across the squash widthwise (shortest distance across) and shred the strands to remove them from the shell.

OVEN METHOD

1.   Preheat the oven to 425°F.

2.   Using a sharp knife, carefully halve the squash lengthwise. Using a spoon or kitchen shears, remove the seeds and strings from the center.

continued

3. In a 9-by-13-inch baking dish filled with ½ inch of water, place each squash half cut-side down. Bake for 40 to 60 minutes until the spaghetti squash shells dent when pushed without mushing (then it's overdone).

4. Using a fork, work across the squash widthwise (shortest distance across) and shred the strands to remove them from the shell.

SLOW COOKER METHOD

1. Using a sharp knife, cut a few slits randomly in the squash and place it in the slow cooker.

2. Cover the cooker and cook on high heat for 3 to 4 hours for a 3- to 4-pound squash. Add 30 minutes for each additional pound you are cooking. The squash is done when you can easily dent it with your finger but it doesn't turn to mush (then it's overdone).

3. Halve the squash lengthwise and, using kitchen shears, cut out the seeds and threads.

4. Using a fork, work across the squash widthwise (shortest distance across) and shred the strands to remove them from the shell.

STORAGE TIP: Freeze the squash strands in a single batch or in individual portions. Thaw in the microwave, or in the refrigerator overnight, and reheat to 165°F.

Per Serving (1 cup spaghetti squash): Calories: 30; Fat: 0g; Carbohydrates: 7g; Fiber: 2g; Protein: 1g; Sodium: 0mg

Marinated Cucumber *and* Tomato Salad

PREP TIME: 15 minutes

This chopped salad won't wilt on you. Even 5 days later, each bite will be as juicy and crunchy as day one. Fresh tomatoes and cucumbers are mixed with Havarti cheese and balsamic glaze for a perfectly portable salad.

3 cups grape
tomatoes, halved

2 English cucumbers,
quartered lengthwise and
cut into ½-inch pieces

4 ounces dill Havarti cheese,
or plain Havarti cheese,
cut into ½-inch dice

1 tablespoon extra-virgin
olive oil

1 tablespoon
balsamic glaze

1 teaspoon chopped
fresh parsley

1 teaspoon garlic powder

½ teaspoon dried oregano

½ teaspoon sea salt

¼ teaspoon dried mint

GLUTEN-FREE • MEDITERRANEAN • SOY-FREE •
VEGETARIAN

In a large bowl, toss together the tomatoes, cucumbers, Havarti, olive oil, balsamic glaze, parsley, garlic powder, oregano, salt, and mint.

NEED MORE CALORIES? Double the amount of cheese.

STORAGE TIP: This recipe is not freezer friendly. Keep refrigerated for 3 to 5 days.

INGREDIENT TIP: Although this recipe is indicated as gluten-free, if this is a concern for you, check the ingredient packaging to ensure all foods were processed in a completely gluten-free facility.

Per Serving (¼ recipe): Calories: 198; Fat: 14g; Carbohydrates: 12g; Fiber: 2g; Protein: 8g; Sodium: 510mg

Teriyaki Eggplant

PREP TIME: 15 minutes | COOK TIME: 18 minutes

Eggplant absorbs the flavors of this soy-ginger marinade for a delicious Asian-inspired grilled summer side dish.

⅓ cup low-sodium
soy sauce

3 tablespoons pure
maple syrup

3 tablespoons sesame oil

1 tablespoon garlic powder

1 tablespoon cornstarch

1½ teaspoons
ground ginger

3 medium eggplant, cut into
1-inch cubes

1 tablespoon sesame seeds

1 scallion, green part
only, sliced

DAIRY-FREE • MEDITERRANEAN • VEGAN

1. In a medium bowl, whisk the soy sauce, maple syrup, sesame oil, garlic powder, cornstarch, and ginger until well combined. Pour the mixture into a large skillet and bring it to a boil over medium heat. Reduce the heat to maintain a simmer and cook for 1 to 2 minutes to thicken.

2. Add the eggplant to the skillet, increase the heat to medium-high, and toss it well to coat. Cook for 10 to 15 minutes, stirring occasionally, or until the eggplant is tender and slightly caramelized.

3. Garnish with sesame seeds and scallion before serving.

NEED MORE CALORIES? Drizzle the eggplant with sesame oil after cooking.

STORAGE TIP: Freeze the eggplant in a single batch or in individual portions. Thaw in the microwave, or in the refrigerator overnight, and reheat to 165°F.

INGREDIENT TIP: To make this recipe gluten-free and soy-free, use coconut aminos instead of the soy sauce.

Per Serving (⅙ recipe): Calories: 171; Fat: 8g; Carbohydrates: 24g; Fiber: 7g; Protein: 4g; Sodium: 611mg

Chinese Five-Spice Bok Choy

PREP TIME: 10 minutes | COOK TIME: 15 minutes

The crisp, delicate taste of bok choy pairs well with soy and other traditional Asian flavors. Its leaves seem to soak up the seasonings as they become more tender and glazed.

1 tablespoon avocado oil

4 garlic cloves, minced

4 baby bok choy, halved lengthwise

¼ cup low-sodium soy sauce

1 teaspoon Chinese five-spice

DAIRY-FREE • MEDITERRANEAN • VEGAN

1.   In a large skillet over medium heat, heat the avocado oil. Add the garlic and sauté for about 1 minute until tender.

2.   Add the bok choy and soy sauce to the skillet and sprinkle with the five-spice seasoning. Cover the skillet and let the bok choy steam for 4 to 5 minutes.

3.   Remove the lid, flip the bok choy, and cook until the liquid evaporates and the bok choy reaches your desired tenderness.

NEED MORE CALORIES? Drizzle the bok choy with sesame oil before serving.

STORAGE TIP: Freeze the bok choy in a single batch or in individual portions. Thaw in the microwave, or in the refrigerator overnight, and reheat to 165°F.

INGREDIENT TIP: To make this recipe gluten-free and soy-free, use coconut aminos instead of the soy sauce.

Per Serving (¼ recipe): Calories: 55; Fat: 4g; Carbohydrates: 3g; Fiber: 1g; Protein: 2g; Sodium: 761mg

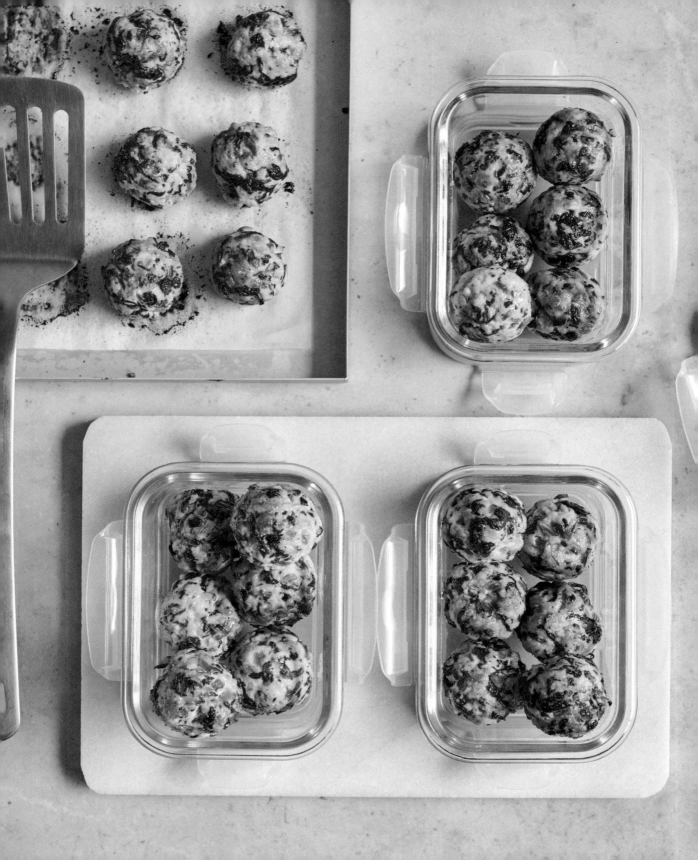

CHAPTER NINE

Satisfying Proteins

Whole Greek Chicken 144

Lemon-Pepper Dill Salmon Foil Packets 146

Skillet Turkey Taco Meat 147

Easy Baked Falafel 148

Easy Shredded Chicken 150

Red Wine–Marinated Steak 151

Lemon, Garlic, and White Wine Shrimp Skillet 152

Salmon Burgers 153

Greek Turkey, Spinach, and Feta Meatballs 154

Crispy and Versatile Baked Tofu 155

« Greek Turkey, Spinach, and Feta Meatballs (page 154)

Whole Greek Chicken

PREP TIME: 1 hour, plus up to 24 hours to marinate | COOK TIME: 1 hour, 30 minutes

Tender, juicy whole chicken roasted in lemon and herbs leaves your house smelling cozy and inviting. This chicken is moist on the inside and crispy and lemony on the outside.

1 (4-pound) whole chicken

1 onion, sliced

¾ cup avocado oil

⅓ cup freshly squeezed
   lemon juice

4 garlic cloves, minced

1 tablespoon dried oregano

1 tablespoon dried parsley

1 teaspoon dried dill

1 teaspoon dried basil

1 teaspoon onion flakes

1 teaspoon sea salt

1 teaspoon dried rosemary

½ teaspoon dried thyme

¼ teaspoon freshly ground
   black pepper

¼ teaspoon dried marjoram

DAIRY-FREE • GLUTEN-FREE • MEDITERRANEAN • SOY-FREE

1.   In a large gallon-size freezer bag, combine the chicken, onion, avocado oil, lemon juice, garlic, oregano, parsley, dill, basil, onion flakes, salt, rosemary, thyme, pepper, and marjoram. Seal the bag, shake to coat, and refrigerate to marinate for 1 to 24 hours.

2.   Preheat the oven to 450°F.

3.   Remove the chicken from the bag and place it in a roasting pan, baking dish, or 10-inch cast iron skillet. Surround the chicken with the sliced onions and pour the marinade over the top.

4.   Roast for 20 minutes.

5.   Reduce the oven temperature to 350°F and roast the chicken for 40 minutes more. Baste the chicken with the drippings every 10 to 15 minutes or so. Toss the onions with drippings each time you baste the chicken. The chicken is done when it reaches an internal temperature of 165°F.

6.   Let the chicken sit for 10 to 30 minutes before carving and serving.

7. To properly carve the chicken:

- Cut between the breast and the legs on each side. Using tongs to hold the legs, pull the breast back away from the legs. Use a knife to cut the skin on the underside of the chicken to separate the legs from the breast fully.

- Separate the legs from the backbone with a knife. Then cut across the leg and thigh joint to separate those pieces.

- Remove the wings from the breast pieces by cutting through the joint.

- Remove the breasts from the breastbone and cut each breast in half.

STORAGE TIP: Freeze the chicken in a single batch or in individual portions. Thaw in the microwave, or in the refrigerator overnight, and reheat to 165°F.

INGREDIENT TIP: Although this recipe is indicated as gluten-free, if this is a concern for you, check the ingredient packaging to ensure all foods were processed in a completely gluten-free facility.

Per Serving (5 ounces, mix of white and dark meat): Calories: 289; Fat: 18g; Carbohydrates: 3g; Fiber: 1g; Protein: 28g; Sodium: 520mg

Lemon-Pepper Dill Salmon Foil Packets

PREP TIME: 5 minutes | COOK TIME: 20 minutes

Salmon is packed with healthy anti-inflammatory omega-3 fatty acids and protein. This salmon comes out moist and flaky with a hint of lemon, pepper, and dill.

2 pounds salmon fillet

1 lemon, halved and 1 half cut into slices

1 teaspoon freshly ground black pepper

¼ cup chopped fresh dill

DAIRY-FREE • DASH • GLUTEN-FREE • MEDITERRANEAN • SOY-FREE

1. Preheat the oven to 400°F.

2. Cut a piece of aluminum foil big enough to create a steamer packet for your fish fillet. You can cut the fillet in half if you need to make two steamer packets, so it fits.

3. Place the salmon in the center of the foil and squeeze the juice from half a lemon on top. Sprinkle with pepper and top with lemon slices. Place the dill on top of the lemon.

4. Close the foil packet by folding up the long ends to meet and folding one side over the other by 1 inch. Roll in the short ends to seal and create a steamer packet.

5. Bake for 20 minutes, or until the fish flakes easily with a fork (with a minimum internal temperature of 145°F).

NEED MORE CALORIES? Double the portions.

STORAGE TIP: Salmon does not taste great when frozen after cooking. Skip freezing this one and serve it within 3 days.

INGREDIENT TIP: Although this recipe is indicated as gluten-free, check the ingredient packaging to ensure all foods were processed in a completely gluten-free facility.

Per Serving (⅛ recipe): Calories: 123; Fat: 5g; Carbohydrates: 1g; Fiber: 0g; Protein: 17g; Sodium: 37mg

Skillet Turkey Taco Meat

PREP TIME: 10 minutes | COOK TIME: 25 minutes

Turkey meat seasoned with traditional taco flavors and tossed with creamy tomato sauce. Perfect for "Taco Tuesday" or as a salad topping any day of the week!

1 tablespoon avocado oil

½ white onion, chopped

2 garlic cloves, minced

2 pounds ground turkey (93% lean)

1 tablespoon chili powder

½ teaspoon paprika

¼ teaspoon sea salt

¼ teaspoon freshly ground black pepper

1 teaspoon ground cumin

¼ teaspoon cayenne pepper

1 (8-ounce) can tomato sauce

DAIRY-FREE • DASH • GLUTEN-FREE • SOY-FREE

1. In a large skillet, heat the avocado oil over medium heat. Add the onion and garlic and cook for about 1 minute until the onion is translucent.

2. Add the ground turkey, chili powder, paprika, salt, black pepper, cumin, and cayenne. Stir well, breaking up the meat with the back of a spoon. Cook for 10 to 15 minutes until the turkey is no longer pink and beginning to brown.

3. Stir in the tomato sauce and simmer for 10 minutes.

NEED MORE CALORIES? Toss the taco meat with avocado oil and top with shredded Mexican cheese.

STORAGE TIP: Freeze the meat in a single batch or in individual portions. Thaw in the microwave, or in the refrigerator overnight, and reheat to 165°F.

INGREDIENT TIP: Although this recipe is indicated as gluten-free, if this is a concern for you, check the ingredient packaging to ensure all foods were processed in a completely gluten-free facility.

Per Serving (⅙ recipe): Calories: 182; Fat: 11g; Carbohydrates: 4g; Fiber: 1g; Protein: 18g; Sodium: 218mg

Easy Baked Falafel

PREP TIME: 1 hour, 15 minutes | COOK TIME: 30 minutes

This classic Middle Eastern dish, a spiced chickpea patty, is typically deep-fried. This version saves hundreds of calories being baked instead of fried. Although you've found this recipe in the protein section, it also provides a decent amount of carbohydrates. It counts for both your protein and carb meal prep.

2 (15.5-ounce) cans chickpeas, rinsed and drained

½ cup chopped fresh parsley leaves

½ cup chopped fresh cilantro leaves

⅓ cup chopped red onion

⅓ cup chickpea flour, plus more as needed

6 garlic cloves, peeled

4 teaspoons freshly squeezed lemon juice

4 teaspoons ground cumin

1 teaspoon ground coriander

1 teaspoon ground cardamom

1 teaspoon sea salt

½ teaspoon cayenne pepper

1 teaspoon baking soda

Nonstick cooking spray

DAIRY-FREE • DASH • GLUTEN-FREE • MEDITERRANEAN • SOY-FREE • VEGAN

1. In a food processor, combine half each of the chickpeas, parsley, cilantro, red onion, flour, garlic, lemon juice, cumin, coriander, cardamom, salt, and cayenne. Pulse until just combined. Do not overprocess or you'll have hummus and not be able to make falafel.

2. Stir in half the baking soda. Add more flour if the mixture does not stick together well enough to form patties.

3. Remove the dough from the processor and repeat steps 1 and 2 with the remaining half of the ingredients. Refrigerate all the dough for 1 hour, or freeze it for 20 to 30 minutes.

4. Preheat the oven to 375°F. Line a baking sheet with parchment paper and lightly coat it with cooking spray.

5.   Form the dough into 2-inch-diameter patties (the recipe makes about 20), no thicker than ¼ inch. Place the patties on the prepared baking sheet.

6.   Bake for 10 to 12 minutes. Carefully flip the patties, spritz them with cooking spray, and bake for 10 to 15 minutes more until thoroughly cooked and lightly browned.

NEED MORE CALORIES? Serve with tzatziki or tahini dressing.

STORAGE TIP: This recipe is freezer friendly. Thaw in the refrigerator overnight or in the microwave. To regain their original crispiness, reheat the falafel patties in the toaster oven at 400°F until hot. If you reheat them in the microwave, they will still be very flavorful and moist, just not as crispy on the outside.

INGREDIENT TIP: Although this recipe is indicated as gluten-free, if this is a concern for you, check the ingredient packaging to ensure all foods were processed in a completely gluten-free facility.

Per Serving (4 patties): Calories: 262; Fat: 4g; Carbohydrates: 44g; Fiber: 12g; Protein: 14g; Sodium: 381mg

Easy Shredded Chicken

PREP TIME: 5 minutes | **COOK TIME:** 3 to 4 hours

This recipe may not be fancy, but it's a meal-prep-for-weight-loss staple you need to know how to make. Chicken breast is a delicious way to add protein to any meal, including salads, wraps, veggie bowls, casseroles, and sandwiches. Shredded chicken breast is healthier than lunch meat, which is highly processed.

2 pounds boneless, skinless chicken breast

4 cups low-sodium chicken broth, or water

DAIRY-FREE • DASH • GLUTEN-FREE • MEDITERRANEAN • SOY-FREE

1. In a slow cooker, combine the chicken breast and chicken broth.

2. Cover the cooker and cook on high heat for 3 to 4 hours, or low heat for 4 to 6 hours, until the chicken breast shreds easily with two forks (removed from the liquid).

STORAGE TIP: Freeze the shredded chicken in a single batch or in individual portions. Thaw in the microwave, or in the refrigerator overnight, and reheat to 165°F.

INGREDIENT TIP: Although this recipe is indicated as gluten-free, if this is a concern for you, check the ingredient packaging to ensure all foods were processed in a completely gluten-free facility.

Per Serving (4 ounces): Calories: 171; Fat: 4g; Carbohydrates: 0g; Fiber: 0g; Protein: 35g; Sodium: 59mg

Red Wine–Marinated Steak

PREP TIME: 1 hour | COOK TIME: 5 to 20 minutes

Steak is an important source of iron and other minerals in our diet. Lean steak should be enjoyed in moderation when following the Mediterranean and DASH diets.

2 pounds flank
   steak, trimmed

1 cup red wine

½ cup low-sodium
   soy sauce

6 garlic cloves, minced

2 tablespoons dried basil

2 bay leaves

DAIRY-FREE

1. In a large resealable plastic bag, combine the steak, wine, soy sauce, garlic, basil, and bay leaves. Seal the bag and refrigerate to marinate for 1 to 24 hours.

2. Preheat the grill to 450°F.

3. Remove and discard the bay leaves. Place the steak on the grill and cook, turning once about halfway through the cooking time, until it reaches a minimum internal temperature of 130°F for rare, 140°F for medium-rare, 155°F for medium, or 165°F for well-done. Cook the steaks one level below your desired doneness, as they will continue to cook in the microwave when you reheat them (but do cook to a minimum temperature of 130°F).

NEED MORE CALORIES? Eat a bigger portion.

STORAGE TIP: Freeze the steak in a single batch or in individual portions. Thaw in the microwave, or in the refrigerator overnight, and reheat to 165°F.

INGREDIENT TIP: To make this recipe gluten-free and soy-free, use coconut aminos instead of the soy sauce.

Per Serving (⅙ recipe): Calories: 193; Fat: 7g; Carbohydrates: 1g; Fiber: 0g; Protein: 25g; Sodium: 679mg

Lemon, Garlic, *and* White Wine Shrimp Skillet

PREP TIME: 15 minutes | COOK TIME: 15 minutes

This one-dish meal features lemon-garlic shrimp simmered in a delicious white wine sauce and sprinkled with fresh herbs.

½ cup avocado oil

8 garlic cloves, minced

⅔ cup dry white wine

2 pounds medium shrimp, tails on, deveined

½ cup chopped fresh parsley

Juice of 1 lemon

Grated zest of 1 lemon

1 teaspoon freshly ground black pepper

1 teaspoon sea salt

1 lemon, cut into wedges

DAIRY-FREE • GLUTEN-FREE • MEDITERRANEAN • SOY-FREE

1. In a very large skillet, heat the avocado oil over medium heat. Add the garlic and sauté for about 1 minute until translucent and tender.

2. Add the white wine and let it simmer for 10 to 15 minutes to reduce by half.

3. Working in batches as needed, add the shrimp. Cook 2 to 3 minutes, flipping once about halfway through the cooking time, until just pink. (If cooking in batches, combine all the shrimp in the skillet when done.)

4. Stir in the parsley, lemon juice, lemon zest, pepper, and salt. Serve with lemon wedges for squeezing.

NEED MORE CALORIES? Make a double batch and eat a larger portion.

STORAGE TIP: Freeze the shrimp in a single batch or in individual portions. Thaw in the microwave, or in the refrigerator overnight, and reheat to 165°F.

INGREDIENT TIP: Although this recipe is indicated as gluten-free, if this is a concern for you, check the ingredient packaging to ensure all foods were processed in a completely gluten-free facility.

Per Serving (⅙ recipe): Calories: 319; Fat: 19g; Carbohydrates: 4g; Fiber: 0g; Protein: 28g; Sodium: 703mg

Salmon Burgers

PREP TIME: 15 minutes | COOK TIME: 15 minutes

Canned salmon is a convenient and inexpensive source of protein and healthy fats. This recipe turns canned salmon into delicious, fresh-tasting salmon burgers that can be served as part of a meal with roasted veggies and a healthy carb, over a salad, in a bun, or frozen for future use.

2 (6-ounce) cans boneless, skinless salmon, drained

¼ cup chickpea flour

¼ cup crumbled feta cheese

1 large egg

1 tablespoon freshly squeezed lemon juice

1 tablespoon dried parsley

1 teaspoon garlic powder

1 teaspoon onion flakes

½ teaspoon ground chipotle pepper

¼ teaspoon freshly ground black pepper

2 tablespoons avocado oil

DASH • GLUTEN-FREE • MEDITERRANEAN • SOY-FREE

1. In a small bowl, combine the salmon, flour, feta cheese, egg, lemon juice, parsley, garlic powder, onion flakes, chipotle pepper, and black pepper. Gently mix. Form the salmon mixture into 6 (3-inch-diameter) patties.

2. In a large skillet over medium heat, heat the avocado oil. Place the salmon patties in the skillet and cook for 5 to 6 minutes per side until hot and slightly browned on both sides, or until they reach an internal temperature of 165°F.

STORAGE TIP: Freeze individual portions wrapped in plastic. Thaw in the microwave, or in the refrigerator overnight, and reheat at 350°F in the oven on a baking sheet, or in the microwave, to 165°F.

INGREDIENT TIP: Although this recipe is indicated as gluten-free, if this is a concern for you, check the ingredient packaging to ensure all foods were processed in a completely gluten-free facility.

Per Serving (1 burger): Calories: 178; Fat: 10g; Carbohydrates: 4g; Fiber: 1g; Protein: 18g; Sodium: 303mg

Greek Turkey, Spinach, *and* Feta Meatballs

PREP TIME: 15 minutes | COOK TIME: 25 minutes

This simple recipe creates moist and juicy turkey meatballs rolled with feta, spinach, and red onion.

Nonstick cooking spray

2 pounds ground turkey (93% lean)

2 (8-ounce) boxes frozen spinach, thawed and squeezed of excess water

1 red onion, chopped (about 2 cups)

⅔ cup crumbled feta cheese

4 garlic cloves, minced

2 teaspoons dried oregano

1 teaspoon sea salt

½ teaspoon freshly ground black pepper

GLUTEN-FREE • MEDITERRANEAN • SOY-FREE

1.   Preheat the oven to 400°F. Line two baking sheets with aluminum foil and coat them with cooking spray.

2.   In a large bowl, combine the turkey, spinach, red onion, feta cheese, garlic, oregano, salt, and pepper. Gently mix. Using a cookie scoop, form the mixture into 48 meatballs and place them, evenly spaced, on the prepared baking sheets (24 meatballs on each sheet). Do not let them touch. Spritz the tops of the meatballs with cooking spray.

3.   Bake for 20 to 25 minutes, switching the baking sheets from top to bottom racks and turning the racks front to back about halfway through the baking time, or until slightly browned and they reach an internal temperature of 165°F.

STORAGE TIP: These meatballs freeze well. Thaw in the microwave, or in the refrigerator overnight, and reheat to 165°F.

INGREDIENT TIP: No turkey? Substitute lean ground chicken or pork. Pork should be enjoyed in moderation on the DASH and Mediterranean diets.

Although this recipe is indicated as gluten-free, if this is a concern for you, check the ingredient packaging to ensure all foods were processed in a completely gluten-free facility.

Per Serving (6 meatballs): Calories: 226; Fat: 12g; Carbohydrates: 5g; Fiber: 2g; Protein: 25g; Sodium: 545mg

Crispy *and* Versatile Baked Tofu

PREP TIME: 35 minutes | COOK TIME: 30 minutes

Tofu is made from condensed soy milk and is a low-calorie source of plant-based protein. Enjoy this garlicky tofu that is crispy on the outside and tender on the inside.

4 (14-ounce) packages
  extra-firm tofu

¼ cup avocado oil

¼ cup cornstarch

4 teaspoons minced garlic

1 teaspoon sea salt

1 teaspoon freshly ground
  black pepper

DAIRY-FREE • DASH • GLUTEN-FREE • VEGAN

1.   Cut the tofu blocks widthwise to make 3 large slabs from each. Place the slabs on a stack of paper towels or a clean kitchen towel. Cover them with more paper towels or another kitchen towel and place a cutting board or sheet pan on top. Add weight, like heavy pots, pans, or cookbooks. Let the tofu drain for 30 minutes.

2.   Preheat the oven to 400°F and line two baking sheets with parchment paper.

3.   Remove the weights and towels and cut the tofu into ½- to ¾-inch-wide cubes.

4.   In a medium bowl, toss together the tofu, avocado oil, cornstarch, garlic, salt, and pepper. Divide the tofu pieces between the prepared baking sheets.

5.   Bake for 15 minutes. Remove the baking sheets from the oven and flip the tofu pieces. Bake for 15 minutes more until the tofu is golden brown and crispy.

STORAGE TIP: Freeze the tofu in portions wrapped in plastic. Thaw in the microwave, or in the refrigerator overnight, and reheat to 165°F.

INGREDIENT TIP: Skip step 1 if you purchase pre-drained tofu.

Per Serving (⅛ recipe): Calories: 242; Fat: 17g; Carbohydrates: 6g; Fiber: 2g; Protein: 20g; Sodium: 303mg

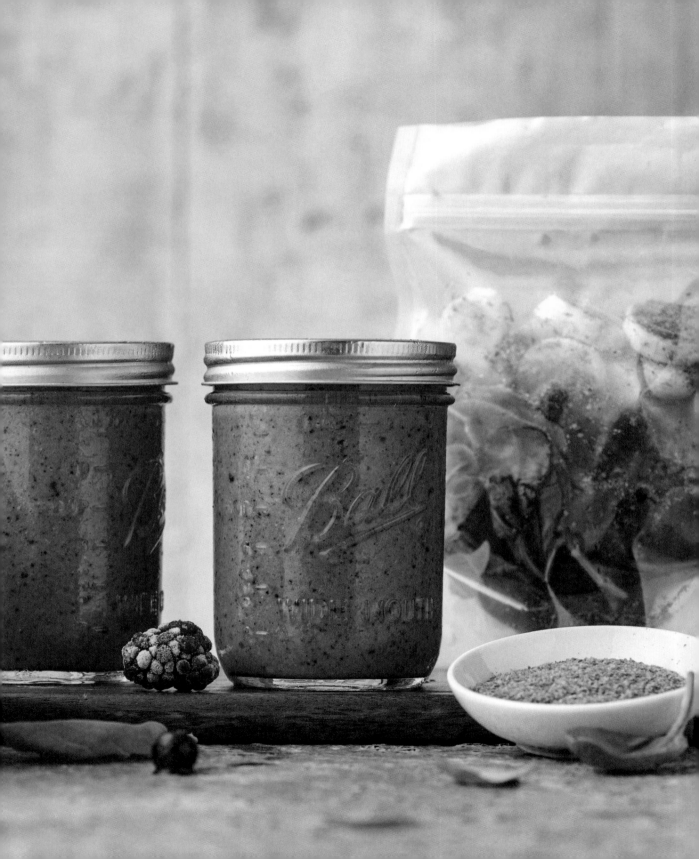

CHAPTER TEN

Snacks

"Kettlecorn" Roasted Chickpeas 158

Hummus-Stuffed Avocado Halves 159

Two-Ingredient Greek Yogurt Hummus Dip and Cucumber 160

Creamy Chocolate Chia Seed Pudding 161

Peanut Butter and Strawberries Yogurt 162

Cottage Cheese Snack Bowls 163

Blueberry Lemon Muffins 164

Meal Prep Smoothie Packs 165

Ham, Cheddar, and Egg Roll-Ups 166

« Meal Prep Smoothie Packs (page 165)

"Kettlecorn" Roasted Chickpeas

PREP TIME: 10 minutes | COOK TIME: 50 minutes

These sweet, salty, crunchy chickpeas will satisfy your urge to crunch and provide you with protein as well as healthy carbs.

2 (15-ounce) cans chickpeas, drained and rinsed

2 teaspoons avocado oil

2 tablespoons pure maple syrup

½ teaspoon sea salt

DAIRY-FREE • DASH • GLUTEN-FREE • MEDITERRANEAN • SOY-FREE • VEGAN

1. Preheat the oven to 425°F. Line a baking sheet with parchment paper.

2. Using a clean kitchen towel, dry the chickpeas and place them in a small bowl. Add the avocado oil and toss to coat. Spread the chickpeas evenly across the prepared baking sheet.

3. Bake for 20 minutes.

4. Drizzle the chickpeas with the maple syrup and season with salt. Toss to combine.

5. Bake for 20 to 30 minutes, tossing every 10 minutes, or until the chickpeas are crunchy.

STORAGE TIP: Store the chickpeas, uncovered, for 3 to 5 days at room temperature. Don't put them in the refrigerator or cover them because they won't stay crunchy!

INGREDIENT TIP: If you aren't feeling the sweet and salty combo, mix up the seasonings but follow the same process. The nutrition info will be the same.

Per Serving (about ⅓ cup roasted chickpeas): Calories: 166; Fat: 4g; Carbohydrates: 27g; Fiber: 6g; Protein: 7g; Sodium: 203mg

Hummus-Stuffed Avocado Halves

PREP TIME: 10 minutes

Don't fear fat! The fat and fiber in avocados help keep you full. Avocados can be a little bland, but they are deliciously creamy. Amp up the flavor with your favorite hummus and a sprinkle of sea salt and cayenne pepper.

Freshly squeezed lime juice, for the avocado halves

3 large avocados, halved and pitted

¾ cup hummus

¼ teaspoon sea salt

¼ teaspoon cayenne pepper (optional)

DAIRY-FREE • DASH • GLUTEN-FREE • MEDITERRANEAN • SOY-FREE • VEGAN

1. Rub the lime juice over the cut side of the avocados to keep them from turning brown.

2. Fill each avocado half with 2 tablespoons of hummus. Sprinkle each with salt and cayenne (if using).

STORAGE TIP: This recipe is not freezer friendly. Keep refrigerated for 3 to 5 days.

INGREDIENT TIP: Although this recipe is indicated as gluten-free, if this is a concern for you, check the ingredient packaging to ensure all foods were processed in a completely gluten-free facility.

Per Serving (½ stuffed avocado): Calories: 234; Fat: 20g; Carbohydrates: 13g; Fiber: 8g; Protein: 4g; Sodium: 236mg

Two-Ingredient Greek Yogurt Hummus Dip *and* Cucumber

PREP TIME: 15 minutes

This recipe seriously amps up the protein content of your hummus, plus adds a bit more creaminess and a slight tang. Perfectly refreshing to dip your veggies in!

6 cucumbers, thinly sliced using a mandoline

1 cup hummus

½ cup plain nonfat Greek yogurt

DASH • GLUTEN-FREE • MEDITERRANEAN • SOY-FREE • VEGETARIAN

1. Divide the sliced cucumbers among 6 storage containers.

2. In a small bowl, stir together the hummus and yogurt. Place ¼ cup of the mixture into each of 6 small storage containers. Refrigerate and serve together.

NEED MORE CALORIES? Mix in ¼ cup extra-virgin olive oil for a creamier, higher-fat snack!

STORAGE TIP: This recipe will keep, refrigerated, for up to 1 week. Do not freeze.

INGREDIENT TIP: Although this recipe is indicated as gluten-free, if this is a concern for you, check the ingredient packaging to ensure all foods were processed in a completely gluten-free facility.

Per Serving (¼ cup dip and 1 cucumber): Calories: 157; Fat: 8g; Carbohydrates: 18g; Fiber: 4g; Protein: 6g; Sodium: 192mg

Creamy Chocolate Chia Seed Pudding

PREP TIME: 4 hours

Chia seeds absorb 12 times their weight in water to create a pudding that is similar to rice pudding in texture but much more nutritious. This pudding is velvety smooth, creamy, and ultra-chocolatey.

3 cups coconut milk
   (from a carton)

1 cup chia seeds

6 scoops collagen powder

½ cup unsweetened
   cocoa powder

¼ cup pure maple syrup

12 drops vanilla stevia

DAIRY-FREE • DASH • GLUTEN-FREE • SOY-FREE

1.   In a large shallow bowl, stir together the coconut milk, chia seeds, collagen powder, cocoa powder, maple syrup, and stevia. Cover the bowl and refrigerate for 4 to 24 hours. (If you don't have a shallow bowl, split this recipe into multiple bowls to chill. If the bowl is too deep, the chia seeds will sink to the bottom and only half the recipe will gel properly.)

2.   Portion ½-cup servings into 6 small Mason jars or other storage containers.

NEED MORE CALORIES? Top the pudding with your favorite nuts or seeds!

STORAGE TIP: Keep the pudding refrigerated for up to 1 week. Freeze the pudding in individual portions and thaw in the refrigerator overnight. Serve cold.

INGREDIENT TIP: Substitute any unflavored protein powder for the collagen powder!

Per Serving (½ cup): Calories: 309; Fat: 13g; Carbohydrates: 31g; Fiber: 11g; Protein: 23g; Sodium: 105mg

Peanut Butter *and* Strawberries Yogurt

PREP TIME: 10 minutes

Greek yogurt with peanut butter is a sweet and creamy high-protein snack that will keep you full for hours. Mix in peanut butter and strawberries for a super-filling snack, breakfast, or dessert.

1½ cups plain nonfat
Greek yogurt

3 tablespoons natural
peanut butter

6 to 7 drops stevia

3 cups fresh strawberries

DASH • GLUTEN-FREE • MEDITERRANEAN • SOY-FREE • VEGETARIAN

In a small bowl, stir together the yogurt, peanut butter, and stevia. Dip the strawberries in the yogurt or cut them up and mix them in for a healthy snack.

NEED MORE CALORIES? Top each serving with granola or honey-roasted peanuts.

STORAGE TIP: Keep refrigerated for up to 3 days. This recipe is not freezer friendly.

INGREDIENT TIP: Although this recipe is indicated as gluten-free, if this is a concern for you, check the ingredient packaging to ensure all foods were processed in a completely gluten-free facility.

Per Serving (½ cup strawberries with ¼ cup dip): Calories: 118; Fat: 6g; Carbohydrates: 11g; Fiber: 2g; Protein: 8g; Sodium: 37mg

Cottage Cheese Snack Bowls

PREP TIME: 10 minutes

These sweet and creamy cottage cheese bowls are a delicious mix of chewy raisins, creamy cottage cheese, salty, crunchy pumpkin seeds, and sweet blueberries drizzled with honey. A delicious before-bed or anytime snack.

3 cups low-fat cottage cheese

6 tablespoons raisins

1½ cups fresh blueberries

½ cup roasted, salted pumpkin seeds

3 tablespoons honey

DASH • GLUTEN-FREE • SOY-FREE • VEGETARIAN

1. Into each of the 6 meal prep containers, place ½ cup of cottage cheese.

2. Top each serving with 1 tablespoon of raisins, ¼ cup of blueberries, a heaping tablespoon of pumpkin seeds, and 1 teaspoon of honey.

NEED MORE CALORIES? Eat double portions!

INGREDIENT TIP: Although this recipe is indicated as gluten-free, if this is a concern for you, check the ingredient packaging to ensure all foods were processed in a completely gluten-free facility.

Per Serving (1 bowl): Calories: 231; Fat: 9g; Carbohydrates: 26g; Fiber: 3g; Protein: 15g; Sodium: 335mg

Blueberry Lemon Muffins

PREP TIME: 15 minutes | **COOK TIME:** 30 minutes

Almond flour is higher in protein and fat than all-purpose flour, so it's more filling and creates a more nutritionally balanced baked good. Enjoy these healthy lemony blueberry muffins for a snack or for breakfast.

Nonstick cooking spray (optional)

2 large eggs

½ cup pure maple syrup

2 teaspoons vanilla extract

2 teaspoons lemon extract

2 cups blanched almond flour

½ teaspoon baking soda

½ teaspoon sea salt

1 cup fresh blueberries

DAIRY-FREE • DASH • GLUTEN-FREE • MEDITERRANEAN • SOY-FREE • VEGETARIAN

1.   Preheat the oven to 350°F. Coat a muffin tin with cooking spray or line it with silicone muffin tin liners.

2.   In a small bowl, whisk the eggs, maple syrup, vanilla and lemon extracts.

3.   Add the almond flour, baking soda, and salt and stir until well combined. Fold in the blueberries. Fill each muffin cup half-way with the batter.

4.   Bake for 25 to 30 minutes, or until a toothpick inserted in the muffins comes out clean.

NEED MORE CALORIES? Top each muffin with almond butter right before you eat it. You could also fold in some walnuts with the blueberries for added calories.

INGREDIENT TIP: Although this recipe is indicated as gluten-free, if this is a concern for you, check the ingredient packaging to ensure all foods, especially oats, were processed in a completely gluten-free facility.

Per Serving (1 muffin): Calories: 136; Fat: 10g; Carbohydrates: 8g; Fiber: 2g; Protein: 5g; Sodium: 163mg

Meal Prep Smoothie Packs

PREP TIME: 15 minutes

These meal prep smoothies are creamy and refreshing, plus you don't have to pull out and put back a million ingredients when you want one.

6 cups frozen mixed berries

3 bananas, peeled
and halved

6 cups fresh spinach

6 tablespoons ground
flaxseed

6 cups low-fat (2%)
milk, divided

DASH • GLUTEN-FREE • MEDITERRANEAN • SOY-FREE • VEGETARIAN

1.   Into each of the 6 quart-size freezer bags, combine 1 cup of berries, ½ banana, 1 cup of spinach, and 1 tablespoon of flax-seed. Press the air from the bags, seal, and freeze.

2.   To make a smoothie, in a high-speed blender, combine the contents of freezer bag and 1 cup of milk and process until smooth.

NEED MORE CALORIES? Add a handful of nuts to each smoothie.

INGREDIENT TIP: Switch up the types of fruit to get different flavors! Pineapple and mango make a delicious combo. Make dairy-free and vegan smoothies using a nondairy milk and ½ scoop unflavored nondairy protein powder.

Although this recipe is indicated as gluten-free, if this is a concern for you, check the ingredient packaging to ensure all foods, especially oats, were processed in a completely gluten-free facility.

Per Serving (1 smoothie): Calories: 314; Fat: 8g; Carbohydrates: 51g; Fiber: 9g; Protein: 14g; Sodium: 164mg

Ham, Cheddar, *and* Egg Roll-Ups

PREP TIME: 5 minutes | **COOK TIME:** 15 minutes

Eggs roll-ups with Black Forest ham and melty Cheddar cheese. You'll love each bite of this savory snack that can be eaten in a flash for a filling high-protein snack.

5 large eggs

Nonstick cooking spray

5 Black Forest ham slices

5 Cheddar cheese slices

DASH • GLUTEN-FREE • SOY-FREE

1.   In a small bowl, beat 1 egg.

2.   Coat an 8-inch nonstick skillet with cooking spray and place it over medium-low heat. When hot enough, the pan should sizzle slightly when water is sprinkled in it.

3.   Add the egg to the skillet, tilting the skillet to allow the egg to fully spread the width of the pan. Cook for 1 minutes until the egg is completely set. Flip the egg and cook for 1 minute more before removing the "egg tortilla" from the skillet. Repeat with the remaining eggs, coating the pan with cooking spray between each one, and let the tortillas cool completely.

4.   Onto each egg tortilla, layer 1 slice of ham and 1 slice of Cheddar cheese. Roll them up. Refrigerate in an airtight container for 3 to 5 days. Eat cold or reheat in the microwave.

NEED MORE CALORIES? Use 2 eggs to make a thicker tortilla and layer on 2 slices of ham instead of 1. For fewer calories, omit the cheese.

STORAGE TIP: Surprisingly, cooked eggs do freeze well. These can be reheated in the microwave from frozen or fresh.

Per Serving (1 roll-up): Calories: 221; Fat: 15g; Carbohydrates: 2g; Fiber: 0g; Protein: 18g; Sodium: 479mg

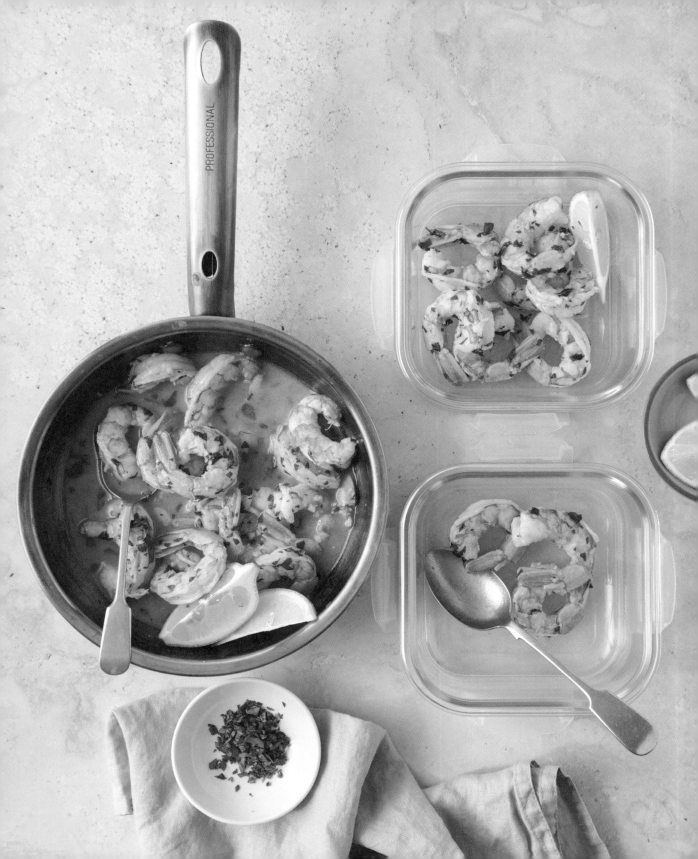

The Dirty Dozen™ and the Clean Fifteen™

A nonprofit environmental watchdog organization called Environmental Working Group (EWG) looks at data supplied by the US Department of Agriculture (USDA) and the Food and Drug Administration (FDA) about pesticide residues. Each year it compiles a list of the best and worst pesticide loads found in commercial crops. You can use these lists to decide which fruits and vegetables to buy organic to minimize your exposure to pesticides and which produce is considered safe enough to buy conventionally. This does not mean they are pesticide free, though, so wash these fruits and vegetables thoroughly. The list is updated annually, and you can find it online at EWG.org/FoodNews.

DIRTY DOZEN™

1. strawberries
2. spinach
3. kale
4. nectarines
5. apples
6. grapes
7. peaches
8. cherries
9. pears
10. tomatoes
11. celery
12. potatoes

†Additionally, nearly three-quarters of hot pepper samples contained pesticide residues.

CLEAN FIFTEEN™

1. avocados
2. sweet corn
3. pineapples
4. sweet peas (frozen)
5. onions
6. papayas
7. eggplants
8. asparagus
9. kiwis
10. cabbages
11. cauliflower
12. cantaloupes
13. broccoli
14. mushrooms
15. honeydew melons

Measurement Conversions

	US STANDARD	US STANDARD (OUNCES)	METRIC (APPROXIMATE)
Volume Equivalents (Liquid)	2 tablespoons	1 fl. oz.	30 mL
	¼ cup	2 fl. oz.	60 mL
	½ cup	4 fl. oz.	120 mL
	1 cup	8 fl. oz.	240 mL
	1½ cups	12 fl. oz.	355 mL
	2 cups or 1 pint	16 fl. oz.	475 mL
	4 cups or 1 quart	32 fl. oz.	1 L
	1 gallon	128 fl. oz.	4 L
Volume Equivalents (Dry)	⅛ teaspoon	———	0.5 mL
	¼ teaspoon	———	1 mL
	½ teaspoon	———	2 mL
	¾ teaspoon	———	4 mL
	1 teaspoon	———	5 mL
	1 tablespoon	———	15 mL
	¼ cup	———	59 mL
	⅓ cup	———	79 mL
	½ cup	———	118 mL
	⅔ cup	———	156 mL
	¾ cup	———	177 mL
	1 cup	———	235 mL
	2 cups or 1 pint	———	475 mL
	3 cups	———	700 mL
	4 cups or 1 quart	———	1 L
	½ gallon	———	2 L
	1 gallon	———	4 L
Weight Equivalents	½ ounce	———	15 g
	1 ounce	———	30 g
	2 ounces	———	60 g
	4 ounces	———	115 g
	8 ounces	———	225 g
	12 ounces	———	340 g
	16 ounces or 1 pound	———	455 g

Index

A

Almond butter
  Make-Ahead Fruit and
    Yogurt Parfaits, 34
Almonds
  Crunchy Roasted Green
    Beans with Slivered
    Almonds, 131
  Customizable Protein
    Steel Cut Oatmeal
    Cups, 117–118
  Make-Ahead Fruit and
    Yogurt Parfaits, 34
Apples
  Portable Breakfast
    Protein Boxes, 61
  Slow-Cooked Pork
    Tenderloin with Apples
    and Carrots, 67–68
Arugula
  Pan-Seared Trout with
    Tzatziki Sauce, Arugula,
    and Quinoa Salad,
    73–74
Asparagus
  Herb-Roasted Asparagus
    and Feta, 130
  steaming, 25
Avocados
  Hummus-Stuffed Avocado
    Halves, 159
  Tuna Salad Wraps, 108

B

Bacon
  Portable Breakfast
    Protein Boxes, 61
Bacon, Canadian
  Meal Prep Breakfast
    Sandwiches, 69–70

Bananas
  Meal Prep Smoothie
    Packs, 165
Beans
  Easy Layered Enchilada
    Casserole, 105–106
  Slow Cooker Three-Bean
    Chili, 79
  Steak Burrito Bowls, 94–95
Beef
  Red Wine–Marinated
    Steak, 151
  Seasoned Ground Beef, 60
  Spicy Tomato-Basil Zoodles
    with Beef, 58–59
  Steak Burrito Bowls, 94–95
  Taco-Stuffed Sweet
    Potatoes, 56–57
Berries
  Blueberry Lemon Muffins, 164
  Caramelized Butternut
    Squash and Farro
    Salad, 124–125
  Cottage Cheese Snack
    Bowls, 163
  Customizable Protein
    Steel Cut Oatmeal
    Cups, 117–118
  Greek Yogurt Blueberry
    Bites, 109
  Make-Ahead Fruit and
    Yogurt Parfaits, 34
  Meal Prep Smoothie
    Packs, 165
  Peanut Butter and
    Strawberries Yogurt, 162
  Protein-Packed Peanut
    Butter and Berry
    Overnight Oats, 53
Beverages, 17

Blueberry Lemon Muffins, 164
Bok Choy, Chinese Five
    Spice, 141
Bowls
  Cottage Cheese Snack
    Bowls, 163
  Steak Burrito Bowls, 94–95
Broccoli
  Custom Mini Quiches, 96–97
  Garlic and Herb Farro
    with Lemon-Pepper
    Broccoli, 50–51
  Meal Prep Breakfast
    Sandwiches, 69–70
  steaming, 25
Brussels sprouts
  Crispy Roasted Garlicky
    Brussels Sprouts, 135
  steaming, 25
Bulk shopping, 19

C

Calories, 4–5, 9
Caprese Chicken Pasta with
    Roasted Tomatoes, 82–83
Caramelized Butternut Squash
    and Farro Salad, 124–125
Carbohydrates, 15, 16
Carrots
  Crunchy Rainbow Salad with
    Thai Peanut Dressing, 75
  Customizable Finger
    Foods Lunch, 35
  Glazed Slow Cooker
    Carrots, 132
  Slow-Cooked Pork
    Tenderloin with Apples
    and Carrots, 67–68
  steaming, 25
  Tuna Salad Wraps, 108

Cashews
  Sheet Pan Sweet and
    Spicy Salmon with
    Veggies, 42–43
Cauliflower
  Roasted Sweet Potatoes
    and Cauliflower, 92–93
  steaming, 25
Celery
  Classic Chicken Salad
    in a Pita, 52
  Muffin Tin Mini Lentil
    Loaves, 126–127
  Tuna Salad Wraps, 108
Cheddar cheese, 166
  Custom Mini Quiches, 96–97
  Meal Prep Breakfast
    Sandwiches, 69–70
Cheese. See specific
Chia seeds
  Creamy Chocolate Chia
    Seed Pudding, 161
  Protein-Packed Peanut
    Butter and Berry
    Overnight Oats, 53
Chicken
  Caprese Chicken Pasta with
    Roasted Tomatoes,
    82–83
  Chopped Rainbow
    Mediterranean
    Salad, 40–41
  Classic Chicken Salad
    in a Pita, 52
  Easy Layered Enchilada
    Casserole, 105–106
  Easy Sheet Pan Chicken
    Fajitas, 71–72
  Easy Shredded Chicken, 150
  Italian Marinated Grilled
    Chicken, 48–49
  One-Pan Crispy Chicken
    Thighs with Roasted
    Red Potatoes and
    Green Beans, 32–33

Sheet Pan Hummus Chicken
    and Zucchini, 98
Slow Cooker BBQ
    Chicken, 91
Slow Cooker
    Garlic-Parmesan
    Chicken, 103
Slow Cooker Three-Bean
    Chili, 79
Whole Greek
    Chicken, 144–145
Chickpeas
  Chopped Rainbow
    Mediterranean
    Salad, 40–41
  Easy Baked Falafel, 148–149
  "Kettlecorn" Roasted
    Chickpeas, 158
Chili, Slow Cooker
    Three-Bean, 79
Chimichurri Shrimp
    Skewers, 107
Chinese Five-Spice
    Bok Choy, 141
Chocolate
  Creamy Chocolate Chia
    Seed Pudding, 161
  Peanut Butter Chocolate
    Energy Balls, 99
Chopped Rainbow
    Mediterranean
    Salad, 40–41
Cinnamon-Roasted Sweet
    Potatoes, 114
Classic Chicken Salad
    in a Pita, 52
Coconut-Lime Brown Rice, 115
Coconut milk
  Coconut-Lime Brown
    Rice, 115
  Creamy Chocolate Chia
    Seed Pudding, 161
Corn
  Easy Layered Enchilada
    Casserole, 105–106

Grilled Chili-Lime
    Fiesta Corn, 123
Cottage cheese
  Cottage Cheese Snack
    Bowls, 163
  High-Protein Egg
    Salad Boxes, 81
Creamy Chocolate Chia
    Seed Pudding, 161
Crispy and Versatile
    Baked Tofu, 155
Crispy Roasted Garlicky
    Brussels Sprouts, 135
Crispy Roasted Greek
    Vegetable Medley,
    133–134
Crunchy Rainbow Salad with
    Thai Peanut Dressing, 75
Crunchy Roasted Green Beans
    with Slivered Almonds, 131
Cucumbers
  Chopped Rainbow
    Mediterranean
    Salad, 40–41
  Marinated Cucumber and
    Tomato Salad, 139
  Mediterranean Lentil Salad
    with Tahini Dressing, 80
  Two-Ingredient Greek
    Yogurt Hummus Dip
    and Cucumber, 160
Customizable Finger
    Foods Lunch, 35
Customizable Protein
    Steel Cut Oatmeal
    Cups, 117–118
Custom Mini Quiches, 96–97

D
Dairy-free
  Blueberry Lemon
    Muffins, 164
  Caramelized Butternut
    Squash and Farro
    Salad, 124–125

Chimichurri Shrimp
   Skewers, 107
Chinese Five-Spice
   Bok Choy, 141
Cinnamon-Roasted Sweet
   Potatoes, 114
Classic Chicken Salad
   in a Pita, 52
Coconut-Lime Brown Rice, 115
Creamy Chocolate Chia
   Seed Pudding, 161
Crispy and Versatile
   Baked Tofu, 155
Crispy Roasted Garlicky
   Brussels Sprouts, 135
Crispy Roasted
   Greek Vegetable
   Medley, 133–134
Crunchy Rainbow Salad with
   Thai Peanut Dressing, 75
Crunchy Roasted Green
   Beans with Slivered
   Almonds, 131
Customizable Protein
   Steel Cut Oatmeal
   Cups, 117–118
Easy Baked Falafel, 148–149
Easy Shredded Chicken, 150
Garlic and Herb Farro
   with Lemon-Pepper
   Broccoli, 50–51
Hummus-Stuffed Avocado
   Halves, 159
Italian Marinated Grilled
   Chicken, 48–49
"Kettlecorn" Roasted
   Chickpeas, 158
Lemon, Garlic, and White
   Wine Shrimp Skillet, 152
Lemon-Pepper Dill Salmon
   Foil Packets, 146
Mixed Herb Smashed Red
   Potatoes, 120–121
Muffin Tin Mini Lentil
   Loaves, 126–127

One-Pan Crispy Chicken
   Thighs with Roasted
   Red Potatoes and
   Green Beans, 32–33
Peanut Butter Chocolate
   Energy Balls, 99
Portable Breakfast
   Protein Boxes, 61
Red Wine–Marinated
   Steak, 151
Roasted Sweet Potatoes
   and Cauliflower,
   92–93
Seasoned Ground Beef, 60
Sheet Pan Hummus Chicken
   and Zucchini, 98
Sheet Pan Sweet and
   Spicy Salmon with
   Veggies, 42–43
Skillet Turkey Taco Meat, 147
Slow-Cooked Pork
   Tenderloin with Apples
   and Carrots, 67–68
Slow Cooker BBQ
   Chicken, 91
Spaghetti Squash, 137–138
Taco-Stuffed Sweet
   Potatoes, 56–57
Tangy and Spicy Perfect
   Plantains, 119
Teriyaki Eggplant, 140
Tuna Salad Wraps, 108
Turkey, Spinach, and Sweet
   Potato Breakfast
   Hash, 84–85
Whole Greek
   Chicken, 144–145
DASH diet, 7
Blueberry Lemon
   Muffins, 164
Caprese Chicken Pasta with
   Roasted Tomatoes, 82–83
Caramelized Butternut
   Squash and Farro
   Salad, 124–125

Chopped Rainbow
   Mediterranean
   Salad, 40–41
Cinnamon-Roasted Sweet
   Potatoes, 114
Classic Chicken Salad
   in a Pita, 52
Coconut-Lime Brown
   Rice, 115
Cottage Cheese Snack
   Bowls, 163
Creamy Chocolate Chia
   Seed Pudding, 161
Crispy and Versatile
   Baked Tofu, 155
Crispy Roasted Garlicky
   Brussels Sprouts, 135
Crispy Roasted
   Greek Vegetable
   Medley, 133–134
Crunchy Roasted Green
   Beans with Slivered
   Almonds, 131
Customizable Protein
   Steel Cut Oatmeal
   Cups, 117–118
Custom Mini Quiches, 96–97
Easy Baked Falafel,
   148–149
Easy Shredded Chicken, 150
Foil Packet Parmesan
   Squash, 136
Garlic and Herb Farro
   with Lemon-Pepper
   Broccoli, 50–51
Glazed Slow Cooker
   Carrots, 132
Greek Yogurt Blueberry
   Bites, 109
Grilled Chili-Lime
   Fiesta Corn, 123
Ham, Cheddar, and Egg
   Roll-Ups, 166
Herb-Roasted Asparagus
   and Feta, 130

DASH diet *(continued)*
  Hummus-Stuffed Avocado
    Halves, 159
  Italian Marinated Grilled
    Chicken, 48–49
  "Kettlecorn" Roasted
    Chickpeas, 158
  Lemon-Pepper Dill Salmon
    Foil Packets, 146
  Make-Ahead Fruit and
    Yogurt Parfaits, 34
  Meal Prep Smoothie
    Packs, 165
  Mediterranean Lentil Salad
    with Tahini Dressing, 80
  Mixed Herb Smashed Red
    Potatoes, 120–121
  Parmesan Polenta
    Rounds, 122
  Peanut Butter and
    Strawberries Yogurt, 162
  Peanut Butter Chocolate
    Energy Balls, 99
  Portable Breakfast
    Protein Boxes, 61
  Protein-Packed Peanut
    Butter and Berry
    Overnight Oats, 53
  Roasted Garlic-Parmesan
    Quinoa, 116
  Roasted Sweet Potatoes
    and Cauliflower, 92–93
  Salmon Burgers, 153
  Seasoned Ground Beef, 60
  Sheet Pan Hummus Chicken
    and Zucchini, 98
  Skillet Turkey Taco Meat, 147
  Slow-Cooked Pork
    Tenderloin with Apples
    and Carrots, 67–68
  Slow Cooker BBQ
    Chicken, 91
  Slow Cooker
    Garlic-Parmesan
    Chicken, 103

  Slow Cooker Three-Bean
    Chili, 79
  Spaghetti Squash, 137–138
  Stuffed Bell Peppers, 104
  Tangy and Spicy Perfect
    Plantains, 119
  Turkey, Spinach, and Sweet
    Potato Breakfast
    Hash, 84–85
  Two-Ingredient Greek
    Yogurt Hummus Dip
    and Cucumber, 160
Drinks, 17

E

Easy Baked Falafel, 148–149
Easy Layered Enchilada
  Casserole, 105–106
Easy Sheet Pan Chicken
  Fajitas, 71–72
Easy Shredded Chicken, 150
Edamame
  Crunchy Rainbow Salad
    with Thai Peanut
    Dressing, 75
Eggplants
  Crispy Roasted
    Greek Vegetable
    Medley, 133–134
  steaming, 25
  Teriyaki Eggplant, 140
Eggs
  Blueberry Lemon Muffins, 164
  Custom Mini Quiches, 96–97
  Ham, Cheddar, and Egg
    Roll-Ups, 166
  High-Protein Egg
    Salad Boxes, 81
  Meal Prep Breakfast
    Sandwiches, 69–70
  Portable Breakfast
    Protein Boxes, 61
  Stuffed Bell Peppers, 104
Equipment, 18
Exercise, 6

F

Farro
  Caramelized Butternut
    Squash and Farro
    Salad, 124–125
  Garlic and Herb Farro
    with Lemon-Pepper
    Broccoli, 50–51
Fats, 16, 17
Feta cheese
  Chopped Rainbow
    Mediterranean
    Salad, 40–41
  Greek Turkey,
    Spinach, and Feta
    Meatballs, 154
  Herb-Roasted Asparagus
    and Feta, 130
  Mediterranean Lentil
    Salad with Tahini
    Dressing, 80
  Salmon Burgers, 153
  Stuffed Bell Peppers, 104
First Five-Day Superefficient
    Prep Plan
  meal plan, 89
  recipes, 91–99
  shopping list, 88
  step-by-step guide, 90
First Flavor Variety
    Five-Day Meal Prep
  meal plan, 65
  recipes, 67–75
  shopping list, 64–65
  step-by-step guide, 66
First Quick and Easy Three-Day
    Meal Prep Plan
  meal plan, 47
  recipes, 48–53
  shopping list, 46
  step-by-step guide, 47
Fish
  Lemon-Pepper Dill Salmon
    Foil Packets, 146

Pan-Seared Trout with
Tzatziki Sauce, Arugula,
and Quinoa Salad,
73–74
Salmon Burgers, 153
Sheet Pan Sweet and
Spicy Salmon with
Veggies, 42–43
Tuna Salad Wraps, 108
Five-Day Breakfast and
Lunch Meal Prep Plan
meal plan, 31
recipes, 32–35
shopping list, 30
step-by-step guide, 31
Five-Day Prep Lunch and
Dinner Meal Plan
meal plan, 37
recipes, 38–43
shopping list, 36
step-by-step guide, 37
Foil Packet Parmesan
Squash, 136
Food safety, 21–22

G

Garlic and Herb Farro
with Lemon-Pepper
Broccoli, 50–51
Genetics, 6
Glazed Slow Cooker
Carrots, 132
Gluten-free
Blueberry Lemon
Muffins, 164
Caramelized Butternut
Squash and Farro
Salad, 124–125
Chimichurri Shrimp
Skewers, 107
Chopped Rainbow
Mediterranean
Salad, 40–41
Cinnamon-Roasted Sweet
Potatoes, 114

Coconut-Lime Brown
Rice, 115
Cottage Cheese Snack
Bowls, 163
Creamy Chocolate Chia
Seed Pudding, 161
Crispy and Versatile
Baked Tofu, 155
Crispy Roasted Garlicky
Brussels Sprouts, 135
Crispy Roasted
Greek Vegetable
Medley, 133–134
Crunchy Roasted Green
Beans with Slivered
Almonds, 131
Customizable Protein
Steel Cut Oatmeal
Cups, 117–118
Custom Mini Quiches, 96–97
Easy Baked Falafel, 148–149
Easy Layered Enchilada
Casserole, 105–106
Easy Sheet Pan Chicken
Fajitas, 71–72
Easy Shredded Chicken, 150
Foil Packet Parmesan
Squash, 136
Garlic and Herb Farro
with Lemon-Pepper
Broccoli, 50–51
Glazed Slow Cooker
Carrots, 132
Greek Turkey, Spinach, and
Feta Meatballs, 154
Greek Yogurt Blueberry
Bites, 109
Grilled Chili-Lime
Fiesta Corn, 123
Ham, Cheddar, and Egg
Roll-Ups, 166
Herb-Roasted Asparagus
and Feta, 130
Hummus-Stuffed Avocado
Halves, 159

Italian Marinated Grilled
Chicken, 48–49
"Kettlecorn" Roasted
Chickpeas, 158
Lemon, Garlic, and White
Wine Shrimp Skillet, 152
Lemon-Pepper Dill Salmon
Foil Packets, 146
Make-Ahead Fruit and
Yogurt Parfaits, 34
Marinated Cucumber and
Tomato Salad, 139
Meal Prep Smoothie
Packs, 165
Mediterranean Lentil Salad
with Tahini Dressing, 80
Mixed Herb Smashed Red
Potatoes, 120–121
One-Pan Crispy Chicken
Thighs with Roasted
Red Potatoes and
Green Beans, 32–33
Pan-Seared Trout with
Tzatziki Sauce, Arugula,
and Quinoa Salad, 73–74
Parmesan Polenta
Rounds, 122
Peanut Butter and
Strawberries Yogurt, 162
Peanut Butter Chocolate
Energy Balls, 99
Portable Breakfast
Protein Boxes, 61
Protein-Packed Peanut
Butter and Berry
Overnight Oats, 53
Roasted Garlic-Parmesan
Quinoa, 116
Roasted Sweet Potatoes
and Cauliflower, 92–93
Salmon Burgers, 153
Seasoned Ground Beef, 60
Sheet Pan Hummus Chicken
and Zucchini, 98
Skillet Turkey Taco Meat, 147

Gluten-free (continued)
Slow Cooker BBQ
Chicken, 91
Slow Cooker Garlic-
Parmesan Chicken, 103
Slow Cooker Spaghetti
Squash Turkey
Bolognese, 38–39
Slow Cooker Three-Bean
Chili, 79
Spaghetti Squash, 137–138
Spicy Tomato-Basil Zoodles
with Beef, 58–59
Steak Burrito Bowls, 94–95
Stuffed Bell Peppers, 104
Taco-Stuffed Sweet
Potatoes, 56–57
Tangy and Spicy Perfect
Plantains, 119
Turkey, Spinach, and Sweet
Potato Breakfast
Hash, 84–85
Two-Ingredient Greek
Yogurt Hummus Dip
and Cucumber, 160
Whole Greek
Chicken, 144–145
Goat cheese
Spicy Tomato-Basil Zoodles
with Beef, 58–59
Greek Turkey, Spinach, and
Feta Meatballs, 154
Greek Yogurt Blueberry
Bites, 109
Green beans
Crunchy Roasted Green
Beans with Slivered
Almonds, 131
One-Pan Crispy Chicken
Thighs with Roasted
Red Potatoes and
Green Beans, 32–33
steaming, 25
Grilled Chili-Lime Fiesta
Corn, 123
Grocery shopping, 19

H
Ham, Cheddar, and Egg
Roll-Ups, 166
Havarti cheese
Customizable Finger
Foods Lunch, 35
Marinated Cucumber and
Tomato Salad, 139
Health considerations, 8
Herb-Roasted Asparagus
and Feta, 130
High-Protein Egg Salad
Boxes, 81
Hummus
Customizable Finger
Foods Lunch, 35
Hummus-Stuffed Avocado
Halves, 159
Sheet Pan Hummus Chicken
and Zucchini, 98
Tuna Salad Wraps, 108
Two-Ingredient Greek
Yogurt Hummus Dip
and Cucumber, 160

I
Italian Marinated Grilled
Chicken, 48–49

K
Kale
Crunchy Rainbow Salad
with Thai Peanut
Dressing, 75
Mediterranean Lentil
Salad with Tahini
Dressing, 80
"Kettlecorn" Roasted
Chickpeas, 158

L
Leftovers, 22–23
Lemon, Garlic, and White Wine
Shrimp Skillet, 152
Lemon-Pepper Dill Salmon
Foil Packets, 146

Lentils
Mediterranean Lentil Salad
with Tahini Dressing, 80
Muffin Tin Mini Lentil
Loaves, 126–127
Lettuce
Steak Burrito Bowls, 94–95
Tuna Salad Wraps, 108

M
Make-Ahead Fruit and
Yogurt Parfaits, 34
Marinated Cucumber and
Tomato Salad, 139
Meal planning and
prepping, 17–18
benefits of, 9–10
efficiency, 20
First Five-Day Superefficient
Prep Plan, 88–99
First Flavor Variety Five-Day
Meal Prep, 64–75
First Quick and Easy
Three-Day Meal
Prep Plan, 46–53
Five-Day Breakfast
and Lunch Meal
Prep Plan, 30–35
Five-Day Prep Lunch and
Dinner Meal Plan, 36–43
1 carb/1 protein/1 veggie, 6
portioning, 21
Second Five-Day
Superefficient Prep
Plan, 100–109
Second Flavor Variety
Five-Day Meal Prep
Plan, 76–85
Second Quick and Easy
Three-Day Meal
Prep Plan, 54–61
storing, 21–22
Meal Prep Breakfast
Sandwiches, 69–70
Meal Prep Smoothie
Packs, 165

Mediterranean diet, 7

Blueberry Lemon
Muffins, 164

Caprese Chicken Pasta
with Roasted
Tomatoes, 82–83

Caramelized Butternut
Squash and Farro
Salad, 124–125

Chimichurri Shrimp
Skewers, 107

Chinese Five-Spice
Bok Choy, 141

Chopped Rainbow
Mediterranean
Salad, 40–41

Cinnamon-Roasted Sweet
Potatoes, 114

Classic Chicken Salad
in a Pita, 52

Coconut-Lime Brown
Rice, 115

Crispy Roasted Garlicky
Brussels Sprouts, 135

Crispy Roasted
Greek Vegetable
Medley, 133–134

Crunchy Rainbow Salad with
Thai Peanut Dressing, 75

Crunchy Roasted Green
Beans with Slivered
Almonds, 131

Customizable Protein
Steel Cut Oatmeal
Cups, 117–118

Easy Baked Falafel, 148–149

Easy Layered Enchilada
Casserole, 105–106

Easy Sheet Pan Chicken
Fajitas, 71–72

Easy Shredded Chicken, 150

Foil Packet Parmesan
Squash, 136

Garlic and Herb Farro
with Lemon-Pepper
Broccoli, 50–51

Glazed Slow Cooker
Carrots, 132

Greek Turkey, Spinach, and
Feta Meatballs, 154

Greek Yogurt Blueberry
Bites, 109

Grilled Chili-Lime
Fiesta Corn, 123

Herb-Roasted Asparagus
and Feta, 130

High-Protein Egg
Salad Boxes, 81

Hummus-Stuffed Avocado
Halves, 159

Italian Marinated Grilled
Chicken, 48–49

"Kettlecorn" Roasted
Chickpeas, 158

Lemon, Garlic, and White
Wine Shrimp Skillet, 152

Lemon-Pepper Dill Salmon
Foil Packets, 146

Marinated Cucumber and
Tomato Salad, 139

Meal Prep Smoothie
Packs, 165

Mediterranean Lentil Salad
with Tahini Dressing, 80

Mixed Herb Smashed Red
Potatoes, 120–121

Muffin Tin Mini Lentil
Loaves, 126–127

One-Pan Crispy Chicken
Thighs with Roasted
Red Potatoes and
Green Beans, 32–33

Pan-Seared Trout with
Tzatziki Sauce, Arugula,
and Quinoa Salad,
73–74

Parmesan Polenta
Rounds, 122

Peanut Butter and
Strawberries Yogurt, 162

Peanut Butter Chocolate
Energy Balls, 99

Portable Breakfast
Protein Boxes, 61

Protein-Packed Peanut
Butter and Berry
Overnight Oats, 53

Roasted Garlic-Parmesan
Quinoa, 116

Roasted Sweet Potatoes
and Cauliflower, 92–93

Salmon Burgers, 153

Sheet Pan Hummus Chicken
and Zucchini, 98

Sheet Pan Sweet and
Spicy Salmon with
Veggies, 42–43

Slow Cooker BBQ Chicken, 91

Slow Cooker
Garlic-Parmesan
Chicken, 103

Slow Cooker Spaghetti
Squash Turkey
Bolognese, 38–39

Slow Cooker Three-Bean
Chili, 79

Spaghetti Squash, 137–138

Stuffed Bell Peppers, 104

Tangy and Spicy Perfect
Plantains, 119

Teriyaki Eggplant, 140

Tuna Salad Wraps, 108

Turkey, Spinach, and Sweet
Potato Breakfast
Hash, 84–85

Two-Ingredient Greek
Yogurt Hummus Dip
and Cucumber, 160

Whole Greek Chicken,
144–145

Mediterranean Lentil
Salad with Tahini
Dressing, 80

Mexican cheese blend

Easy Layered Enchilada
Casserole, 105–106

Easy Sheet Pan Chicken
Fajitas, 71–72

Mexican cheese blend
(continued)
Slow Cooker Three-Bean
Chili, 79
Steak Burrito Bowls, 94–95
Mixed Herb Smashed Red
Potatoes, 120–121
Mozzarella cheese
Caprese Chicken Pasta with
Roasted Tomatoes, 82–83
Custom Mini Quiches, 96–97
Slow Cooker Spaghetti
Squash Turkey
Bolognese, 38–39
Muffins, Blueberry Lemon, 164
Muffin Tin Mini Lentil
Loaves, 126–127
Mushrooms
Custom Mini Quiches, 96–97
Slow Cooker
Garlic-Parmesan
Chicken, 103
Slow Cooker Spaghetti
Squash Turkey
Bolognese, 38–39

O

Oats
Customizable Protein
Steel Cut Oatmeal
Cups, 117–118
Muffin Tin Mini Lentil
Loaves, 126–127
Peanut Butter Chocolate
Energy Balls, 99
Protein-Packed Peanut
Butter and Berry
Overnight Oats, 53
Oaxaca cheese
Grilled Chili-Lime
Fiesta Corn, 123
One-Pan Crispy Chicken
Thighs with Roasted
Red Potatoes and
Green Beans, 32–33

P

Pan-Seared Trout with Tzatziki
Sauce, Arugula, and
Quinoa Salad, 73–74
Parmesan cheese
Foil Packet Parmesan
Squash, 136
Parmesan Polenta
Rounds, 122
Roasted Garlic-Parmesan
Quinoa, 116
Slow Cooker
Garlic-Parmesan
Chicken, 103
Pasta, Caprese Chicken
with Roasted
Tomatoes, 82–83
Peanut butter
Crunchy Rainbow Salad
with Thai Peanut
Dressing, 75
Peanut Butter and
Strawberries Yogurt, 162
Peanut Butter Chocolate
Energy Balls, 99
Portable Breakfast
Protein Boxes, 61
Protein-Packed Peanut
Butter and Berry
Overnight Oats, 53
Peppers
Chopped Rainbow
Mediterranean
Salad, 40–41
Crispy Roasted
Greek Vegetable
Medley, 133–134
Customizable Finger
Foods Lunch, 35
Custom Mini Quiches,
96–97
Easy Sheet Pan Chicken
Fajitas, 71–72
High-Protein Egg
Salad Boxes, 81

Slow Cooker Three-Bean
Chili, 79
Stuffed Bell Peppers, 104
Plantains, Tangy and
Spicy Perfect, 119
Plate method, 4–5, 14
Polenta Rounds,
Parmesan, 122
Pork. See also Bacon; Ham
Slow-Cooked Pork
Tenderloin with Apples
and Carrots, 67–68
Portable Breakfast
Protein Boxes, 61
Portion size, 21
Potatoes. See also
Sweet potatoes
Mixed Herb Smashed Red
Potatoes, 120–121
One-Pan Crispy Chicken
Thighs with Roasted
Red Potatoes and
Green Beans, 32–33
Produce, 15
Protein, 14, 17
Protein-Packed Peanut
Butter and Berry
Overnight Oats, 53
Pumpkin seeds
Caramelized Butternut
Squash and Farro
Salad, 124–125
Cottage Cheese Snack
Bowls, 163

Q

Quinoa
Easy Sheet Pan Chicken
Fajitas, 71–72
Pan-Seared Trout with
Tzatziki Sauce, Arugula,
and Quinoa Salad,
73–74
Roasted Garlic-Parmesan
Quinoa, 116

R

Raisins
  Cottage Cheese Snack
    Bowls, 163
Recipes, about, 8, 24–25
Red Wine–Marinated Steak, 151
Reheating, 23–24
Resting metabolic rate
    (RMR), 5, 9
Rice
  Chimichurri Shrimp
    Skewers, 107
  Coconut-Lime Brown
    Rice, 115
  Sheet Pan Hummus Chicken
    and Zucchini, 98
  Slow Cooker
    Garlic-Parmesan
    Chicken, 103
Roasted Garlic-Parmesan
    Quinoa, 116
Roasted Sweet Potatoes and
    Cauliflower, 92–93

S

Salads
  Caramelized Butternut
    Squash and Farro
    Salad, 124–125
  Chopped Rainbow
    Mediterranean
    Salad, 40–41
  Classic Chicken Salad
    in a Pita, 52
  Crunchy Rainbow Salad
    with Thai Peanut
    Dressing, 75
  Marinated Cucumber and
    Tomato Salad, 139
  Mediterranean Lentil Salad
    with Tahini Dressing, 80
  Pan-Seared Trout with
    Tzatziki Sauce, Arugula,
    and Quinoa Salad, 73–74

Salmon
  Lemon-Pepper Dill Salmon
    Foil Packets, 146
  Salmon Burgers, 153
  Sheet Pan Sweet and
    Spicy Salmon with
    Veggies, 42–43
Sandwiches and wraps
  Classic Chicken Salad
    in a Pita, 52
  Ham, Cheddar, and Egg
    Roll-Ups, 166
  Meal Prep Breakfast
    Sandwiches, 69–70
  Salmon Burgers, 153
  Tuna Salad Wraps, 108
Sausage
  Slow Cooker Spaghetti
    Squash Turkey
    Bolognese, 38–39
  Turkey, Spinach, and Sweet
    Potato Breakfast
    Hash, 84–85
Seasoned Ground Beef, 60
Second Five-Day
    Superefficient Prep Plan
  meal plan, 101
  recipes, 103–109
  shopping list, 100
  step-by-step guide, 102
Second Flavor Variety
    Five-Day Meal Prep Plan
  meal plan, 77
  recipes, 79–85
  shopping list, 76–77
  step-by-step guide, 78
Second Quick and Easy
    Three-Day Meal Prep Plan
  meal plan, 55
  recipes, 56–61
  shopping list, 54
  step-by-step guide, 55
Sheet Pan Hummus Chicken
    and Zucchini, 98

Sheet Pan Sweet and
    Spicy Salmon with
    Veggies, 42–43
Shrimp
  Chimichurri Shrimp
    Skewers, 107
  Lemon, Garlic, and White
    Wine Shrimp Skillet, 152
Skillet Turkey Taco Meat, 147
Slow-Cooked Pork Tenderloin
    with Apples and
    Carrots, 67–68
Slow Cooker BBQ Chicken, 91
Slow Cooker Garlic-Parmesan
    Chicken, 103
Slow Cooker Spaghetti Squash
    Turkey Bolognese, 38–39
Slow Cooker Three-Bean
    Chili, 79
S.M.A.R.T. goals, 14
Smoothie Packs, Meal
    Prep, 165
Soy-free
  Blueberry Lemon
    Muffins, 164
  Caprese Chicken Pasta with
    Roasted Tomatoes, 82–83
  Caramelized Butternut
    Squash and Farro
    Salad, 124–125
  Chimichurri Shrimp
    Skewers, 107
  Chopped Rainbow
    Mediterranean
    Salad, 40–41
  Cinnamon-Roasted Sweet
    Potatoes, 114
  Classic Chicken Salad
    in a Pita, 52
  Coconut-Lime Brown
    Rice, 115
  Cottage Cheese Snack
    Bowls, 163
  Creamy Chocolate Chia
    Seed Pudding, 161

Soy-free *(continued)*

Crispy Roasted Garlicky Brussels Sprouts, 135

Crispy Roasted Greek Vegetable Medley, 133–134

Crunchy Roasted Green Beans with Slivered Almonds, 131

Customizable Finger Foods Lunch, 35

Customizable Protein Steel Cut Oatmeal Cups, 117–118

Custom Mini Quiches, 96–97

Easy Baked Falafel, 148–149

Easy Layered Enchilada Casserole, 105–106

Easy Sheet Pan Chicken Fajitas, 71–72

Easy Shredded Chicken, 150

Foil Packet Parmesan Squash, 136

Garlic and Herb Farro with Lemon-Pepper Broccoli, 50–51

Glazed Slow Cooker Carrots, 132

Greek Turkey, Spinach, and Feta Meatballs, 154

Greek Yogurt Blueberry Bites, 109

Grilled Chili-Lime Fiesta Corn, 123

Ham, Cheddar, and Egg Roll-Ups, 166

Herb-Roasted Asparagus and Feta, 130

High-Protein Egg Salad Boxes, 81

Hummus-Stuffed Avocado Halves, 159

Italian Marinated Grilled Chicken, 48–49

"Kettlecorn" Roasted Chickpeas, 158

Lemon, Garlic, and White Wine Shrimp Skillet, 152

Lemon-Pepper Dill Salmon Foil Packets, 146

Make-Ahead Fruit and Yogurt Parfaits, 34

Marinated Cucumber and Tomato Salad, 139

Meal Prep Breakfast Sandwiches, 69–70

Meal Prep Smoothie Packs, 165

Mediterranean Lentil Salad with Tahini Dressing, 80

Mixed Herb Smashed Red Potatoes, 120–121

One-Pan Crispy Chicken Thighs with Roasted Red Potatoes and Green Beans, 32–33

Pan-Seared Trout with Tzatziki Sauce, Arugula, and Quinoa Salad, 73–74

Parmesan Polenta Rounds, 122

Peanut Butter and Strawberries Yogurt, 162

Peanut Butter Chocolate Energy Balls, 99

Portable Breakfast Protein Boxes, 61

Protein-Packed Peanut Butter and Berry Overnight Oats, 53

Roasted Garlic-Parmesan Quinoa, 116

Roasted Sweet Potatoes and Cauliflower, 92–93

Salmon Burgers, 153

Seasoned Ground Beef, 60

Sheet Pan Hummus Chicken and Zucchini, 98

Skillet Turkey Taco Meat, 147

Slow Cooker BBQ Chicken, 91

Slow Cooker Garlic-Parmesan Chicken, 103

Slow Cooker Spaghetti Squash Turkey Bolognese, 38–39

Slow Cooker Three-Bean Chili, 79

Spaghetti Squash, 137–138

Spicy Tomato-Basil Zoodles with Beef, 58–59

Steak Burrito Bowls, 94–95

Stuffed Bell Peppers, 104

Taco-Stuffed Sweet Potatoes, 56–57

Tangy and Spicy Perfect Plantains, 119

Tuna Salad Wraps, 108

Turkey, Spinach, and Sweet Potato Breakfast Hash, 84–85

Two-Ingredient Greek Yogurt Hummus Dip and Cucumber, 160

Whole Greek Chicken, 144–145

Spaghetti Squash, 137–138

Spicy Tomato-Basil Zoodles with Beef, 58–59

Spinach

Classic Chicken Salad in a Pita, 52

Greek Turkey, Spinach, and Feta Meatballs, 154

Meal Prep Smoothie Packs, 165

Turkey, Spinach, and Sweet Potato Breakfast Hash, 84–85

Squash

Caramelized Butternut Squash and Farro Salad, 124–125

Foil Packet Parmesan
Squash, 136
Slow Cooker Spaghetti
Squash Turkey
Bolognese, 38–39
Spaghetti Squash, 137–138
Stanley, Edward, 8
Starch, 15, 16
Steak Burrito Bowls, 94–95
Storage, 21–22
Stuffed Bell Peppers, 104
Sugar snap peas, 25
Sweet potatoes
Cinnamon-Roasted Sweet
Potatoes, 114
Roasted Sweet Potatoes
and Cauliflower, 92–93
Taco-Stuffed Sweet
Potatoes, 56–57
Turkey, Spinach, and Sweet
Potato Breakfast
Hash, 84–85
Swiss cheese
Custom Mini Quiches, 96–97

T

Taco-Stuffed Sweet
Potatoes, 56–57
Tangy and Spicy Perfect
Plantains, 119
Teriyaki Eggplant, 140
Tofu, Crispy and Versatile
Baked, 155
Tomatoes
Caprese Chicken Pasta with
Roasted Tomatoes, 82–83
Chopped Rainbow
Mediterranean
Salad, 40–41
Easy Layered Enchilada
Casserole, 105–106
Marinated Cucumber and
Tomato Salad, 139
Mediterranean Lentil Salad
with Tahini Dressing, 80

Slow Cooker Three-Bean
Chili, 79
Spicy Tomato-Basil Zoodles
with Beef, 58–59
Tools, 18
Trout, Pan-Seared with Tzatziki
Sauce, Arugula, and
Quinoa Salad, 73–74
Tuna Salad Wraps, 108
Turkey
Customizable Finger
Foods Lunch, 35
Greek Turkey, Spinach, and
Feta Meatballs, 154
Skillet Turkey Taco Meat, 147
Slow Cooker Spaghetti
Squash Turkey
Bolognese, 38–39
Slow Cooker Three-Bean
Chili, 79
Turkey, Spinach, and Sweet
Potato Breakfast
Hash, 84–85
Two-Ingredient Greek
Yogurt Hummus Dip
and Cucumber, 160

V

Vegan
Caramelized Butternut
Squash and Farro
Salad, 124–125
Chinese Five-Spice
Bok Choy, 141
Cinnamon-Roasted Sweet
Potatoes, 114
Coconut-Lime Brown
Rice, 115
Crispy and Versatile
Baked Tofu, 155
Crispy Roasted Garlicky
Brussels Sprouts, 135
Crispy Roasted
Greek Vegetable
Medley, 133–134

Crunchy Roasted Green
Beans with Slivered
Almonds, 131
Customizable Protein
Steel Cut Oatmeal
Cups, 117–118
Easy Baked Falafel, 148–149
Hummus-Stuffed Avocado
Halves, 159
"Kettlecorn" Roasted
Chickpeas, 158
Mixed Herb Smashed Red
Potatoes, 120–121
Muffin Tin Mini Lentil
Loaves, 126–127
Peanut Butter Chocolate
Energy Balls, 99
Roasted Sweet Potatoes
and Cauliflower, 92–93
Spaghetti Squash, 137–138
Tangy and Spicy Perfect
Plantains, 119
Teriyaki Eggplant, 140
Vegetables, 15, 16. See
also specific
High-Protein Egg
Salad Boxes, 81
Sheet Pan Sweet and
Spicy Salmon with
Veggies, 42–43
steaming, 25
Vegetarian. See also Vegan
Blueberry Lemon
Muffins, 164
Cottage Cheese Snack
Bowls, 163
Crunchy Rainbow Salad with
Thai Peanut Dressing, 75
Custom Mini Quiches, 96–97
Foil Packet Parmesan
Squash, 136
Glazed Slow Cooker
Carrots, 132
Greek Yogurt Blueberry
Bites, 109

Vegetarian *(continued)*
Grilled Chili-Lime
Fiesta Corn, 123
Herb-Roasted Asparagus
and Feta, 130
High-Protein Egg
Salad Boxes, 81
Make-Ahead Fruit and
Yogurt Parfaits, 34
Marinated Cucumber and
Tomato Salad, 139
Meal Prep Smoothie
Packs, 165
Mediterranean Lentil Salad
with Tahini Dressing, 80
Parmesan Polenta
Rounds, 122
Peanut Butter and
Strawberries Yogurt, 162
Protein-Packed Peanut
Butter and Berry
Overnight Oats, 53

Roasted Garlic-Parmesan
Quinoa, 116
Stuffed Bell Peppers, 104
Two-Ingredient Greek
Yogurt Hummus Dip
and Cucumber, 160
Visceral fat, 6

W
Weight loss, 4–5
Whole Greek Chicken,
144–145

Y
Yogurt, Greek
Greek Yogurt Blueberry
Bites, 109
Make-Ahead Fruit and
Yogurt Parfaits, 34
Peanut Butter and
Strawberries
Yogurt, 162

Two-Ingredient Greek
Yogurt Hummus Dip
and Cucumber, 160

Z
Zucchini
Chimichurri Shrimp
Skewers, 107
Crispy Roasted
Greek Vegetable
Medley, 133–134
Easy Layered Enchilada
Casserole, 105–106
Foil Packet Parmesan
Squash, 136
Sheet Pan Hummus Chicken
and Zucchini, 98
Slow Cooker
Garlic-Parmesan
Chicken, 103
Spicy Tomato-Basil Zoodles
with Beef, 58–59

Acknowledgments

I want to thank my husband, Paul, who is affectionately known to many of my blog readers as "Mr. Hungry." I could have never completed this book without you.

Thank you to my mom for encouraging me to pursue my dreams and never letting me slack off.

Thank you to my aunt for giving feedback on my vegetarian recipes and for watching your grandnephew while I tested those vegetarian recipes again and again.

I want to thank my in-laws, Marianne, Kal, Megan, and Elizabeth. Thank you to Marianne and Kal for the endless support and encouragement. Thank you to Megan for helping with all the tasks on my blog while I wrote this book. Thank you to Elizabeth for giving me my first tripod and teaching me about food photography.

Thank you to all my blog readers and nutrition clients who encouraged me to keep blogging and posting recipes.

Most importantly, I want to thank God because, without God, I wouldn't be able to do any of this.

About the Author

Kelli Shallal is a Registered Dietitian in private practice with a master's degree in Public Health from Loma Linda University and a National Academy of Sports Medicine Certified Personal Trainer. She is the author behind the popular healthy living blog, Hungry Hobby, and owner of healthy meal planning company, What to Eat? Meal Plans. Kelli's quotes and recipes have been featured on major media outlets including *Today's Dietitian*, *Food & Nutrition Magazine*, *Good Morning Arizona* (3TV), *AZTV*, *Shape*, *Fitness*, *Health*, *Runner's World*, and *Self*.

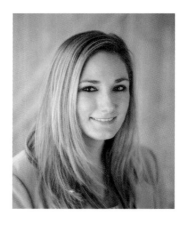

Kelli lives in Phoenix, Arizona, with her husband, Paul, young son, Kal, Rhodesian Ridgeback pup, Nala, and cat, Missy. Find out more about Kelli on her blog www.hungryhobby.net and follow her on Instagram @hungryhobbyrd.